PETER BURWASH'S AEROBIC WORKOUT BOOK FOR MEN

PETER BURWASH'S

AEROBIC WORKOUT BOOK FOR MEN

by Peter Burwash and John Tullius

Photographs by Bruce Haase

DODD, MEAD & COMPANY   New York

Published by Dodd, Mead & Company, Inc.
79 Madison Avenue, New York, N.Y. 10016

Distributed in Canada by
McClelland and Stewart Limited, Toronto

Manufactured in the United States of America
Designed by Joan Greenfield
First Edition

Library of Congress Cataloging in Publication Data
Burwash, Peter.
Peter Burwash's Aerobic workout book for men.
Includes bibliographical references.
1. Aerobic exercises.   2. Exercise for men.   3. Diet.
I. Tullius, John.   II. Title.   III. Title: Aerobic workout book for men.
RA781.15.B87   1984   613.7′1′088041   84-1684
ISBN 0-396-08380-3 (pbk.)

DEDICATION

To Bruce Haase, whose loyalty, determination, and professionalism have inspired me and everyone he's touched.

CONTENTS

FOREWORD

Peter Burwash and I first met on a tennis court. I was unlucky enough to draw him as an opponent in the first round of a tournament in Hawaii. Since he was a world-class player and I was not, since he'd played Davis Cup for Canada, was their number-one player in 1971, and ranked number one in Hawaii in 1973, 1975, and 1977, I knew I was going to lose the match. What I expected was a spectacular display of shots and strategy that would wipe me off the court posthaste. But that didn't happen. Oh, I lost in quick order, to be sure. But instead of great tennis, what beat me, what in fact overwhelmed me, was an unbelievable display of energy. Burwash ran down every ball, climbed the fence to retrieve an overhead, dove for balls, rolled, got up, dove again, and hit a winner. He barely worked up a sweat, wasn't breathing hard, and throughout the match had an eager, bouncing, indefatigable energy.

I had to know how he did it.

Peter Burwash is easily the busiest and most productive man I've ever met. He sleeps three hours a day—four if he's feeling overworked. For the last four years he has averaged one and a quarter million air miles per year. He is president of Peter Burwash International (PBI), the largest international network of tennis professionals in the world, staffing over sixty of the most prestigious tennis clubs and resorts on four continents—in Tokyo, Bangkok, Honolulu, and Houston, for instance.

Peter Burwash has been a worldwide spokesman on health, fitness, and diet for the last fifteen years. He studied physiology at the University of Toronto and the University of Alberta and was named "the most fit person in Canada" after testing at the renowned Percival's Fitness Institute in Toronto. He has been intensively involved with aerobics for many years and has trained his entire staff of professionals to conduct his aerobic workout in PBI resorts around the world.

In addition, Peter tours some two hundred days a year with the Peter Burwash International Tennis Show, which has been described as the Harlem Globetrotters of tennis. The Tennis Show has performed in ninety-four countries, every Canadian province, and all fifty states—for Prince Rainier in Monte Carlo, for Emperor Hirohito's birthday in Tokyo's National Stadium, and at the U.S. Open Tennis Championships for CBS.

Peter also manages a prodigious tour of speaking engagements. He's been the featured speaker at just about every important tennis teachers' conference, including the USTA National Tennis Teachers' Conference held in New York every year during the U.S. Open. And year after year he has spoken at most of the important health and fitness gatherings worldwide—including the National Health Federation, the Total Fitness Conference in Honolulu, and the World Vegetarian Conference.

By now you're probably asking yourself the same question I asked Peter the first day we met: "Where does one person get all that energy?"

Read on if you want to find out.

John Tullius
February 1984

ACKNOWLEDGMENTS

Thanks to Mary Ann Rovai, Lynn Harvey, H. B. Laski, and Shannon Tullius for their tireless efforts in helping us put the manuscript together and to Gene Watanabe for his advice and concern.

A special thank you to Chris Reid whose editing skills have made my words make sense.

INTRODUCTION

WHY DO WE NEED AN AEROBICS WORKOUT BOOK FOR MEN?

One day I met a friend while I was out jogging. When I said, "I didn't know you ran," he answered, "I'm trying to get in shape for my wife's aerobics class."

In the past how often would you have heard a man admit that he had to get in shape before *he* could exercise with his wife? It's always been the other way around. But we're in a new era now.

Aerobics has brought America to its feet. And for good reason. Following a regular, well-planned aerobics exercise program can improve your cardiovascular fitness—which means you'll have a healthier heart. Since heart disease is the number-one killer in this country, simply by maintaining cardiovascular fitness you will have eliminated your main health enemy. And aerobics is the way to do it. People who have a high level of cardiovascular fitness are three times less likely to develop heart disease. A trained heart provides more fuel to the tissues of the body more efficiently. Consequently, it lasts longer.

The first aerobics class I ever attended, back in the late 70's, was a real shock for me. On my left was a fifty-two-year-old woman and on my right was a woman seven months pregnant. After the eight-minute warm-up, I was wiped out. Sweat was pouring off me from the stretching exercises alone. Then they started the aerobics, and after five minutes my tongue was hanging out. And they kept up this grueling pace for an hour.

The expectant mother next to me was carrying an extra twenty-five pounds and yet she was bouncing, kicking high—thoroughly enjoying herself. All I kept thinking was, "Please, no more leg lifts!"

Then they started the floor exercises, and I knew I couldn't go on. But I did. My male ego kept me going. If a fifty-two-year-old woman and a pregnant woman could smile and laugh their way through all this, they'd have to carry me out on a stretcher. And they almost did.

I went to that first aerobics class out of curiosity. There was so much talk about exercising to music that I just had to see what all the fuss was about. But I wasn't all that attracted to the idea of aerobics at first. Basically, I hate to exercise. Now don't get me wrong; I'd play competitive sports all day long, if I could. In fact, all the exercise I ever did was in order to play a sport better. I didn't care about fitness; I just wanted to make the team. But after three years of high school football, I really grew to hate calisthenics. One, two, three, four . . . It's boring and it hurts and there's no thrill of victory—only the agony of sore muscles.

But the major reason I stayed away from aerobics was I wasn't convinced that dancing around to music could get me in shape. Like most men, I had the wrong idea about aerobics.

Women took the right road—the road to health and fitness—when they took to aerobics with so much enthusiasm and in such great numbers. At the same time, aerobics has been done a great disservice by having been branded an almost exclusively female activity. Like diet soft drinks, the image of aerobics is that it's for women. A man drinks beer and plays golf or softball, but he doesn't put on a pair of leotards and dance around to disco music.

And then there are those X-rated aerobics shows on cable television with scantily clad women in heavy make-up exercising to suggestive music. No wonder men think these exercises weren't meant for them.

That's sad, because men in this country desperately need the benefits an aerobics program can offer. Not only can it get you healthy and fit, but it's fun, practical, and convenient. You can do it at home, on the road, in your office, in a hotel room. And you don't have to have a lot of fancy equipment or belong to an expensive health club.

But until now no one had come up with an aerobics workout that was designed to fit the needs and tastes of a man. There is a big difference between well-planned aerobic workouts for men and women. First, a man's fitness needs are different than a woman's. As men gain weight, they tend to deposit the weight in the front of their bodies, particularly around the stomach. A woman's fat usually collects in the back of the body, especially the buttocks and thighs. Men get a "spare tire"; women get "cellulite." Second, men have 20 percent more muscle and 30 percent less essential fat (the fat the body uses, in most part, to cushion the vital organs) than women.

Aerobic workouts such as "jazzercise" and "aerobic dancing" do not allow for these physiological differences between men and women. They are meant to develop and slim a woman's body, and, in the books describing these programs, all the photos and anatomical references are of women.

But perhaps the most important difference is psychological. The exercises in most aerobic workouts rely predominantly on dance steps or dance exercises, and one of the major reasons aerobics caught on with women is that most of them are not embarrassed to dance. But they are put off by the boring calisthenics men seem to like. Aerobics was a nice way of luring women into exercise.

Most men, on the other hand, are embarrassed by the thought of dancing without a partner. So how do we lure the men? First, by developing an aerobics program just for them. Although the exercises in this book are accompanied by suggested music to heighten enjoyment and minimize boredom, the Aerobic Workout for Men is *not* a dance class. It is a series of stretches, aerobic conditioning exercises, and strength exercises developed specifically for the needs and tastes of a man. There is also an emphasis on chest and upper-body strength, areas almost totally ignored in aerobic workouts for women.

Peter Burwash's Aerobic Workout Book for Men is the only book of aerobic exercises specifically designed for men. It will help you strengthen and tone your entire body by just following one of the three different workouts explained: the Get-in-Shape, the Advanced, and the Super workouts. They are tailored to your particular fitness needs —whether you're just getting back into exercising after a long layoff, or you're getting ready for the Olympics.

The Aerobic Workout for Men is all you need to achieve total fitness. There are no complicated point systems to determine if you've gotten enough exercise, such as you find in some books. Nor is there the boredom or the risk of injury as with jogging and weight lifting. And you don't have to participate in several different activities (for example, racquetball, running, and swimming) to ensure that you're getting a complete aerobic workout.

The Aerobic Workout for Men requires no expensive equipment, facilities, or court, and you can do it anywhere, anytime, without a partner. Whether you're a fifty-year-old executive who wants to get back in shape or a top athlete preparing for the rigors of competition, the Aerobic Workout for Men is the ideal exercise program for men. It's easy and convenient to do. Everybody has twenty minutes a day to spend on the program, and this investment of time will give you a solid foundation of health for your whole life.

PART ONE

WHAT'S SO GOOD ABOUT THE GOOD LIFE?

CHAPTER 1

WE'VE GOTTEN OURSELVES INTO A BIG MESS

I Wouldn't Be Caught Dead in a Bathing Suit

I was at the Princess Hotel in Alcapulco when I realized I had to write this book. As a participant at a convention for the Pacific Area Travel Association, I'd spent most of the week meeting, talking to, and getting to be friends with many of the men and women at the convention. In a few days we were a close-knit group; there wasn't anyone I didn't like and a few I knew would be my friends for a lifetime. But by the shape that most of these folks were in, I wasn't sure how long that lifetime would be.

One morning I was sitting at the pool reading a magazine when I saw a huge stomach go by. I looked up and realized it was Neal, a friend I'd made at the convention. Dressed in loose slacks and a Hawaiian shirt, he didn't *look* that fat. But he was! He was carrying at least seventy pounds of excess fat, and it was going to put him in an early grave.

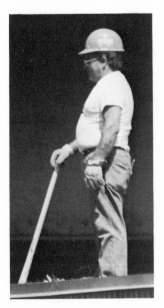

After that I sat there and counted the men at the pool. In two hours, 126 came out in their bathing suits and 126 were overweight. Every single one had a pot belly.

The sad truth is that most Americans don't exercise. Oh, we talk a good game and we swear we're going to get out there and play tennis three or four times a week or run a few miles every day or two. But we don't.

In 1980, The President's Council on Physical Fitness stated that "only about thirty-seven percent of our population exercises on a regular basis (two or three times a week) and sixty-two percent are overweight."[1] That means that nearly two-thirds of our population, over 100 million people, don't jog or play tennis or handball or swim vigorously even twice a week.

Many experts are convinced that the situation is even worse than the President's Council has suggested. For example, Dr. Paul Lessick, an exercise physiologist, believes that only 5 percent of Americans do the kind of exercise that would improve their physical fitness. Dr. Elsworth R. Buskirk, director of the Noll Laboratory for Human Performance Research at Penn State University, believes that only about 5 percent of Americans actually follow a regular exercise program.[2] And Dr. Joseph Ahrends, a cardiologist who specializes in preventive medicine, is even more skeptical. He says that "past the age of thirty-five less than two percent of American males and less than one percent of American females are physically fit."[3]

Sitting by the side of the pool in Alcapulco that morning, I knew they were right.

The Modern Trap

Our modern life-style is chiefly to blame for the pitiful shape most of us are in. Dr. Jean Mayer, a world-famous nutritionist, concurs: "I am convinced that inactivity is the most important factor explaining the frequency of 'creeping' overweight in modern societies. Our bodies' regulation of food intake was just not designed for the highly mechanized condition of modern life. . . . Adapting to these conditions without developing obesity means either that the individual will have to step up his activity or that he will be mildly or acutely hungry all his life."[4]

No people have ever been as pampered as Americans are today. We are so used to riding in automobiles that most of us refuse to walk two blocks to the corner market. Machines mow our lawns and wash our dishes and our clothes. Dirt on our rugs and leaves on our driveways are sucked up by vacuums. Switches, keys, knobs, and buttons do all our work.

Even our play is largely mechanized. We give our golf carts, speedboats, dune buggies, motorcycles, and snowmobiles the workouts while we remain sedentary. And every time we add another "convenience" to our life, we add an inch to our waist. Did you know that, according to Charles Kuntzleman, the national director of the YMCA Fitness Finders Program, if you add an extension phone to your house, you'll also add two pounds per year because you will walk about seventy miles less that year!

This problem is fairly recent. The caveman survived because he could handle himself physically. He ran and fought and foraged in order to survive. If he had decided to spend a day at the beach lying in the sun, it probably would have been his last.

Even as recently as the early twentieth century, Americans got plenty of exercise in the course of their daily lives. They walked nearly everywhere—to the store, to their jobs, to church. They shoveled snow, they raked leaves, they cut their own wood, and they washed their clothes by hand.

It has been only in the last sixty-five years that our exercise habits have begun to change dramatically. Our modern technological society, with its machines and computers, has left us with nothing to do. Instead of walking, we drive; instead of climbing stairs, we ride elevators; instead of playing baseball or basketball, we watch someone else play on television—with a remote control unit so we don't even have to move from our chair.

But what's worse is that this is the way we want it to be. This sedentary approach to life is our ideal, the so-called "good life" we all strive so hard to attain. The solid, hard-working guy is an admirable character, but it's the white-collar worker with a briefcase who retires at forty-five—a man who can afford to hire others to do all the hard work for him—toward which most of us aspire.

Unfortunately, this pursuit of the good life has created a death trap for us. Our sedentary life-style has contributed to a variety of illnesses that affect our vigor, our health, and our productivity. We carry around weight that makes us sag by midday, and we're short of breath after

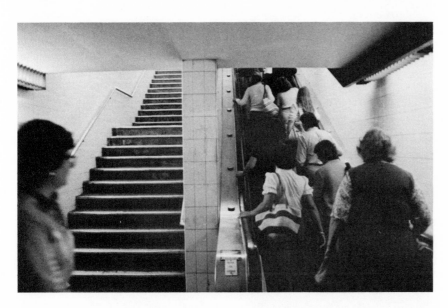

lugging the groceries up a flight of stairs. Our personal confidence and psychological well-being are undermined because we don't feel we look our best.

But, most important of all, this slow physical decline threatens our lives the way plagues once threatened our ancestors. A million of us die every year from heart disease—mostly because at least half of our adult population is more than 25 percent overweight. The list of ailments directly attributable to lack of exercise is staggering—diabetes, depression, gastrointestinal complications, and cardiovascular deterioration just for starters.

I'm not condemning all of modern life. The advancements in medicine and science *have* made our lives more enjoyable, more livable. But you can't ignore the evils of all this progress. We've gotten ourselves into a mess and we're going to have to make some serious adjustments.

And we'd better start now, before it's too late.

CHAPTER 2

HOW I GOT FAT

Never Look to the Rear; It Might Be Gaining on You

Like most kids, I was very active physically. I played football, hockey, and tennis in high school, and tennis and hockey for the University of Toronto.

After college I joined the professional tennis circuit. I was probably the fittest player on the circuit, but that didn't mean much. I was really a hockey player who'd had enough of the brutality of that sport and had decided to pursue my second love—tennis. Since I had a lot to learn as a player and I was competing against the best, I had to try ten times harder than any one else just to survive. So I ran, dove for balls, climbed the fences chasing shots, and ran and ran and ran some more.

I had a deal with my practice partner, Richard Hawkes, to run as much as possible in our practice sessions. If the ball hit the net, we'd both run to the net to pick it up; then back to the baseline to hit again. I knew nothing about aerobics at the time, but I instinctively knew that this nonstop running was the way to get in shape and stay in shape.

And was I ever in shape! Almost everyone on the circuit agreed that I was the fastest and fittest player from 1968 through 1974. That's how I managed to win enough money to stay on the circuit for seven years.

Is That Your Waist Size or Your Age?

Very often when a man hits thirty-five or so and begins to succeed in his profession, he stops exercising. As he moves along in his career or up the corporate ladder, his time becomes less and less his own. I fell into the same trap myself. As soon as I became president of my own company, I had almost no free moment to myself. All my time was dictated by responsibilities to other people. Consequently, exercise came last—which, inevitably, meant not at all.

My mind was constantly stimulated, but my body was turning soft. I had played forty to forty-five tennis tournaments a year for the previous seven years, and suddenly I was playing a half a dozen at the most. The demands of putting together an international business venture were gobbling up all my time and energy. I would go on the road for two or three weeks, during which I wouldn't run a yard or hit a ball. This went on for four or five years before it began to show in my waist. I started getting fat at about twenty-nine because my muscles were turning to fat, but I didn't get a big stomach until I was about thirty-four.

My waistline was in a race with my age to see who was going to get to thirty-six first. And my waistline was winning.

When You Put Me Next to Ralph, I Don't Look That Fat

Before I knew it, I quickly lost the shape and muscle tone I had enjoyed my whole life. I wasn't too concerned yet because I did what we all do—I compared myself to all those guys around me and thought, "Hey, I'm in pretty good shape!"

The problem is that everyone else is in such pitiful shape, it makes you think you're fit. You go to work and see Ralph at the desk next to you; he weighs 250 pounds and his stomach looks like a watermelon. He's carrying around a hundred extra pounds, and you're only forty pounds overweight, so you think you're not doing so bad.

The problem is that we never test ourselves. We never run as far as fifty yards because we know we'd be gasping for breath after twenty-five and that might tell us something we don't want to hear. So we play a little golf on the weekend and we figure we're not *that* out of shape.

We hang onto our illusion of fitness as long as we can. Sure, it's difficult to know the early signs of our body's disintegration—the bloodstream clogged with cholesterol or the muscle tissue filling with fat. The only real measure we have is when our waist expands from thirty-two inches to thirty-four to thirty-six to thirty-eight. When our waist size exceeds our chest size, we know we're in trouble.

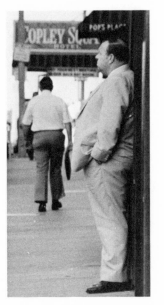

Do You Suck in Your Gut When You Look in the Mirror?

I was about to board a plane from Tonga to Fiji when a huge man approached the check-in desk. I immediately thought, "I wonder what that guy weighs?" That was the first thing the girl at the desk asked him.

"Four hundred and twenty-five pounds," he answered.

"Well," she told him, "you can go first and your baggage can come on the next flight in two days. Or you can send your baggage first. But you can't go together."

Another time, I was in a New York subway and a very overweight woman got stuck in a turnstile. She struggled for several moments before a man who was even bigger than she was came over and pushed her through, to the cheers of a couple hundred people.

Incidents like these show you how much some people are burdened by their excess baggage.

When I was very young my junior high school teacher gave our class a very memorable lesson on how much a little extra baggage can burden you. Every day for five days he tested each member of the class for fitness. We did bench jumps, pushups, situps, running in place, and the classic step test.

After the first two days, we tested in the morning while wearing five-pound belts. We also had to wear the belts for the rest of the day. As the day wore on, we grew more and more physically exhausted, until the belt felt as if it weighed twenty-five pounds. During the last class of the day I could hardly keep my eyes open.

On the fifth day, we tested in the morning without the weight belts and in the afternoon with them. The results showed that our average performance dropped by 20 to 25 percent with the belts on.

At the end of the fifth day, our teacher stood up and said, "Okay, remember this lesson your whole life. Even five pounds can affect your life drastically. Your body may adjust so that it doesn't feel the extra five pounds, but it's there, believe me, and you will only be aware of it when you take that load off your back. Now, think what it would be like if you gained twenty-five pounds."

The adjustments that the body makes when it gains twenty, thirty, or forty pounds are not positive ones. The body doesn't get stronger so it can carry around all that weight more easily. Instead, it tells you that you've got to do *less*. You walk up the stairs more slowly; or your body tells you not to climb those stairs at all.

There are all kinds of subtle adjustments you make when you gain weight. Do you drive around in a parking lot for ten minutes to find a parking space that's a hundred yards closer to the entrance? Do you wear your shirts out to hide your pot? Do you suck your gut in when you look in the mirror?

I know I did. And before I knew it, I was fat. But I was determined to do something about it.

CHAPTER 3

TURNING YOUR LIFE AROUND

It's Time to Have a Long Talk with Yourself

Because our body has been given to us, we don't seem to value it that much. We treat it the way spoiled children treat their toys. Oh, we want to be fit. But most of us don't want to spend the time to get in shape.

There comes a day in nearly every man's life when he looks in the mirror and sees his youth slipping away. His chin has dropped, his skin is sagging, his waist is expanding. Perhaps you play a little tennis with your son and after ten minutes you've had it. Suddenly, you realize it's time to shape up.

Unfortunately, many people have been convinced that there is a quick and easy way to go from fatness to fitness. We care more about looking good, about covering up the flab, than about getting rid of it. So we spend millions on hair transplants, suntan clubs, stomach girdles, and slimming suits. Meanwhile, we've added a chin or two.

Well, it's time to sit down and have a long talk with yourself. Just how much fat are you actually carrying around? Take out a picture album and look at yourself when you were twenty. Were you thin and healthy? Then there's no reason you cannot maintain that weight. Who says you have to get fatter as you get older?

The Best Life Insurance You'll Ever Have

The benefits of exercise are undeniable. A physically fit person is less susceptible to both injury and disease. He can better withstand heat,

11

cold, and fatigue without serious consequences. He also suffers less from nervous tension, constipation, indigestion, and insomnia.

But exercise doesn't just help improve your physical fitness. It affects every facet of your life. Physical activity can make you feel healthier, happier, and younger. A firm, healthy body can make you more attractive, and as your image and self-confidence increase, you'll be more likely to become a participator. You may get a momentary thrill when your favorite football team scores a touchdown, but you'll get a more lasting one when you accomplish something yourself.

In short, exercise is the most efficient, valuable life insurance policy you could ever get.

There Are No Excuses

Of course, we all have a million excuses why we don't exercise regularly: we don't have time, we're too old, we're always on the road, or jogging and calisthenics are just plain boring. And you know how impossible it is to book a tennis court these days.

But there are no good excuses for not following a regular exercise program, because it is your health that's at stake. Sure, the notion of a lifetime commitment scares most of us silly, but it's a necessity. Exercise *must* be a part of your life. It is not a fad.

If you don't exercise, you're hurting yourself. It's that simple! And the first step toward fitness and health is to forget all the excuses and start exercising now!

PART TWO

UNDERSTANDING AEROBICS

CHAPTER 4

A HEALTHY HEART IS THE FOUNDATION OF HEALTH

Everything Revolves Around the Heart

Your health revolves around the health of your heart. You can go blind, lose a leg, even slip into a coma, and you'll live. But when the heart goes, you go. It's that simple.

Heart disease accounts for 40 percent of this country's deaths from all causes, including accidents, murders, suicides, and all other diseases and illnesses. Twenty-four million people suffer from coronary heart disease, and one million die from it each year. Ten percent of all deaths, male and female, before age thirty-five are caused by heart disease.

If you add the other blood-circulation diseases—strokes, arteriosclerosis, and hypertension—half of the deaths in the United States today are from cardiovascular disease. Because of this, our life expectancy, for the first time in over two hundred years, is going down. We aren't living as long as we used to.

These statistics alone should tell you that you've got to get your cardiovascular system in top working order if you want to avoid heart disease.

There is little doubt that infections, heredity, age, smoking, alcohol, and diet contribute to cardiac problems. But lack of cardiovascular exercise is the chief cause.

Have you ever seen an arm or a leg after it's been immobilized for a few months in a cast? It's withered from disuse. The muscles have atrophied from lack of work. And that's only after a few months! Most of us have spent the last *twenty years* avoiding exercise—immobilizing our entire bodies.

The heart responds to inactivity exactly the way the muscles in our legs and arms do. The heart is the muscle engine of our body, and through lack of exercise, through disuse, this engine weakens until all we can do is sputter along like a burnt-out old heap.

There have been many studies that have confirmed the importance of exercise for a healthy heart. A U.S. Public Health Service study, for example, found that sedentary men over the age of thirty-five had coronary attacks almost twice as often as men who were just *moderately* active.[5]

In 1967, 3,263 men were tested to compare the amount of physical activity in their occupations with their frequency of heart disease. Those men with jobs classified as physically demanding had one-third fewer heart attacks than those men with less physically demanding jobs.[6]

In 1973, Dr. J. N. Morris, of the London School of Hygiene and Tropical Medicine, studied the effects of recreational exercise on the hearts of men who had occupations that involved sedentary or very light work. He chose this group because he felt these types of occupations more truly reflected our modern life-styles. As Dr. Morris put it, "Work in advanced societies is increasingly light and sedentary, so any future contribution to public health can only come from exercise taken in leisure time."[7]

His testing clearly showed: "In men recording vigorous exercise the relative risk of developing coronary disease was about a third that in comparable men who did not, and in men reporting much of it still less. Vigorous exercise apparently protected against rapid fatal heart attacks and other first clinical attacks of coronary disease alike, throughout middle age."[8]

In short, people who have physically active occupational and recreational lives have a much lower incidence of heart attacks than those who don't. And the studies cited above only dealt with physical activity in general.

If You Want to Be Hercules—Fine. But You Still Won't Be Healthy unless Your Heart Is

There are five important elements for total physical fitness: cardiovascular fitness, a good body-fat ratio, flexibility, muscular endurance, and muscular strength. By far, the most important of these is cardiovascular fitness.

The basic foundation of health is cardiovascular fitness—a healthy heart. You can look like Hercules; you can throw weights around as if they were made of Styrofoam; you can have a body that makes women swoon—but if you're not cardiovascularly fit, you're not healthy.

The Aerobic Workout for Men is primarily concerned with improving your cardiovascular fitness, your body-fat ratio, and your flexibility. Muscular endurance and strength are given secondary attention. I don't ignore the development of your muscles, though. In fact, I've included muscle-building exercises in the "Workout" section. But my primary consideration is to give you a solid foundation of health, a healthy heart.

Cardiovascular Fitness, Body-Fat Ratio, and Flexibility

Though I will deal with cardiovascular fitness, body-fat ratio, and flexibility in thorough detail in later chapters, I want to briefly define them here.

Cardiovascular fitness refers to the ability of the heart, circulatory system, and lungs to deliver vital oxygen to the cells in every part of the body. The better your cardiovascular fitness, the better you can handle just about every daily task, from cooking breakfast to changing a tire. But, more important, you will be better able to handle high-stress situations and emergencies (such as financial problems or family crises), which could lower your resistance to illness or even lead to a heart attack.

Body-fat ratio refers to the proportion of body fat to body weight. You need some body fat for normal health. It provides protection for your internal organs, keeps the body warm, and is the supply depot from which your body taps its energy. Too much body fat, however, is unhealthy.

The ideal body-fat ratio for men is around 15 percent. (For women it's slightly higher.) When a man's body-fat ratio rises above the 15- to 20-percent level, most fitness and health experts agree he is too fat —even though standard height-weight charts consider ratios much higher than this to be normal. But your height to weight ratio is not an accurate gauge of your fat content because everyone's muscular development is different and your muscles contribute significantly to how much you weigh. For example, a heavily muscled man who is six feet tall could weigh as much as 220 pounds and yet have a body-fat ratio of less than 10 percent. His lean muscles are denser than fat and therefore weigh more than fat. On the other hand, a person who never exercises can appear slim and yet, in fact, carry too much fat. And that's dangerous!

Flexibility is defined as the range of movement of the joints. Degree of flexibility varies from person to person. Gymnasts and dancers, due to their practice routine, have a great deal of flexibility, but everyone needs a reasonable amount of flexibility to perform normal daily activities. Poor flexibility contributes to back pain, muscle pulls, and a variety of ligament and joint problems.

Muscular Endurance and Muscular Strength

Muscular strength refers to the amount of force your muscles can exert at one time. In other words, how much weight can you lift or how high can you jump? But you don't have to be a weight lifter or a high jumper to need strong muscles. Taking the garbage cans out to the curb, rearranging the furniture, and jacking up the car are everyday chores that require sound muscular development. Inadequate muscular strength can lead to strains, pulls, and skeletal problems such as bad posture.

Muscular endurance, on the other hand, refers to the length of time you can do a certain task. If your arms fatigue after you do a few pushups, your muscular endurance is poor. If you're a salesman and you can't stand on your feet all day, you're in trouble.

It's possible, in fact, to have good muscular strength and poor muscular endurance. It's common for a body builder not to be able to run around the block. Often a heavyweight boxer can knock out a gorilla but after three rounds his arms are so tired he can barely lift them.

Muscular strength and endurance can probably be developed best through weight training, but there are many effective and convenient ways to develop your muscles without weights.

Richard A. Berger of Temple University explains: "It doesn't matter whether you overload with weights, with an isokinetic device, through isometrics, or calisthenics. The important thing is to overload the muscles. . . . Muscles don't have eyes. To increase strength, you've got to use heavy weight resistance, and there are several ways to do that. You can use barbells, cables, your own body weight, a towel, or a rope. It really doesn't matter as long as you provide enough resistance."[9]

For those who want to develop their physiques, as well as upper-body and lower-body strength, probably nothing can match a good weight-training program. There are some very strong limitations to weight training, however. First and most important, it does *not* promote cardiovascular fitness. Dr. Kenneth Cooper, "the father of aerobics," explains further:

The weight lifter, or those who emphasize isometrics or calisthenics, represent muscular fitness. These types, who have the right motive but the wrong approach, are stuck with the myth that muscular strength or agility means physical fitness. This is one of the great misconceptions in the field of exercise. The muscles that show—the skeletal muscles—are just one system in the body, and by no means the most important. If your exercise program is directed only at the skeletal muscles, you'll never achieve real physical fitness. [10]

He goes on to say that weight training "builds agility, coordination and muscular strength, particularly in the upper torso. Aerobics builds basic fitness and endurance. A highly conditioned person needs both." [11]

I have included a section in the workout to help you develop muscular strength. But if you want to look like Hercules, you're reading the wrong book. There are dozens of body-building manuals you can consult.

Besides attracting women, the only thing that overdeveloped muscles are going to do for you is allow you to lift things no one else can —which is great if you're a full-time piano mover. But what good does it do a guy to be able to lift three hundred pounds over his head when he's got fifty pounds on his gut and he suffers a coronary in his forties? You can't lift your own casket!

CHAPTER 5

WHY IS AEROBIC EXERCISE THE BEST EXERCISE I CAN DO?

What Do You Mean by Aerobics?

The key to a well-conditioned body is the circulation of oxygen-rich blood. No part of your body can survive without a constant supply of blood from the heart and lungs. The circulatory system is your lifeline. And following a well-planned aerobic workout on a regular basis is the best way to take good care of your cardiovascular and respiratory systems.

Aerobics literally means "air," but even more specifically it means the oxygen in the air. Aerobic exercises all have one thing in common: by making you work at a steady but vigorous pace for an extended period of time (usually between twelve and thirty minutes), they stimulate your heart and lungs and, thereby, demand plenty of oxygen.

Jogging, swimming, and cycling are typical aerobic exercises. But aerobics can be anything that involves the larger muscles of the body and is performed continuously for at least twelve minutes. Also, it must be done at a pace vigorous enough to stimulate the heart so that it beats at around 80 percent of your maximum heart rate. If you exercise according to these guidelines (which I will explain in greater detail later in the book), then your circulatory and respiratory systems will improve and your body fat will be burned—the two main physiological goals of any well-planned aerobics exercise program.

The Body's Need for Oxygen

To understand how to meet your particular energy needs, it's important to understand how energy is manufactured in the body.

The first source of energy that your muscles tap comes from adenosine triphosphate, ATP, a chemical substance made in the muscles almost exclusively by carbohydrates and fat. ATP is the fuel our systems use for strenuous exercise of short duration, because no oxygen is needed for its metabolism. This is called anaerobic exercise ("without oxygen"), and can be performed only in short bursts. (After that, muscles will function efficiently only when oxygen is present.) So you can run a fifty-yard dash all out and not really take a breath.

If this rapid energy consumption lasts for more than a few brief moments, the muscles begin to burn phosphocreatine, PC, which can instantly generate ATP. But even your supplies of PC will only keep you going at top speed for a few extra minutes.

Then the body's second line of energy kicks in with glycogen. Glycogen is made by the body from sugar glucose and stored in limited amounts in the liver and muscles. When the ATP and PC are depleted, glycogen is metabolized in the muscles to produce ATP. This is also an anaerobic reaction.

When your glycogen stores are depleted, the body taps into its third source of energy, which comes from the metabolism of stored fats and carbohydrates. This supply can be almost unlimited. The metabolism of fats and carbohydrates is an *aerobic* reaction, which means it takes more time and lots of oxygen to produce this energy. Thus, the weekend jock will huff and puff after only a few minutes of tough exercise because his body is not conditioned to take in the large supply of oxygen needed to metabolize these fats and carbohydrates for energy. After his stores of ATP and PC are shot, so is he.

The Lungs Are the First Obstacle to Fitness

Simply put, all physical activity requires energy. Your body produces energy by burning food in the presence of oxygen. The body needs energy constantly for all of its functions, from eating to running to thinking. And the blood carries the fuel for energy continuously from the lungs and digestive system to every cell in the body. This process continues nonstop even while you sleep. That's why you must breathe constantly to bring in oxygen (the burning agent that converts fuel to energy).

The problem is that the body can store food as fat but it has no storehouse for oxygen. Therefore, the lungs must constantly feed oxygen into the bloodstream, where the heart pumps the oxygen-rich blood cells to every part of the body.

The first obstacle to oxygen intake, then, is the lungs. In order to be cardiovascularly fit, you must have a healthy respiratory system, because the lungs bring the oxygen into the body. No matter how healthy your heart and bloodstream are, they will not be able to supply the needs of your cardiovascular system if you don't get adequate oxygen into your lungs. The lungs and the cardiovascular system, therefore, work hand in hand and so do the aerobic exercises that develop them.

When you run five miles, you develop the lungs as you develop the heart. Air is forced in and out of the lungs, just as blood is being forcibly pumped in and out of the heart. Because a well-conditioned man has trained the muscles around his lungs to do more work, and has built up the capacity of his lungs, he has the ability to inhale more air for greater lengths of time.

Aerobic Exercise Increases Your Intake of Oxygen

Getting oxygen to the body's tissues, then, is the basis of fitness. The harder you work a muscle, the more oxygen it needs. But the oxygen that an individual can deliver to his muscles depends on how fit his lungs and heart are. He can only burn as much oxygen for muscular energy as he is capable of taking in. Therefore, his "maximum oxygen intake" (the maximum quantity of oxygen a person can take in and transport to his muscles and other tissues while exercising) is the best measure of his fitness.

If a person's heart and lungs—his means of delivery—are so weak that his body's demands for energy surpass his ability to supply it, he's out of shape.

The main physiological objective of an aerobics program is to increase your maximum oxygen intake. Proper aerobic exercise makes your heart beat faster, your lungs expand to take in greater volumes of oxygen, and your blood vessels open up to increase circulation. In short, you are building your body's ability to bring in and transport oxygen throughout your body.

Dr. Kenneth Cooper elaborates on this point: "Aerobics increases maximal oxygen consumption by increasing the efficiency of the means of supply and delivery. In the very act of doing so, it is improving the overall condition of the body, especially its most important parts, the lungs, the heart, the blood vessels and the body tissue, building a bulwark against many forms of illness and disease."[12]

Aerobic exercise makes the muscles work hard enough to force a lot of oxygen through the cardiovascular and respiratory systems. But the exercise is not so intense that the heart and lungs can't handle the body's need for oxygen.

In order for you to get your heart and lungs in shape with aerobics, exercises of enough intensity must be performed for an extended length of time. Chasing after a bus or lifting some boxes at work won't do it. You must do exercises that use up large amounts of oxygen without creating a large oxygen debt. Exercises that leave you gasping for air, such as a sprint, are not aerobic.

CHAPTER 6

IF FAT IS THE KILLER OF THE HEART, WHY DON'T I JUST GO ON A DIET?

Overweight or Overfat?

There are three types of body fat. *Subcutaneous fat,* which makes up 50 percent of your body fat, is that layer of fat that lies directly under the skin. *Deposit fat* is distributed according to each person's hereditary background; it makes up 40 percent of your body fat. *Essential fat* cushions the vital organs of your body from damage and makes up about 10 percent of your body fat. A person can reduce subcutaneous fat and deposit fat, but not essential fat.

Some body fat is necessary to our health because it provides us with internal protection, warmth, and storehouses of energy. But too much body fat is unhealthy.

The more fat a person carries around, the more body tissue his heart must supply with blood. Each pound of fat a person gains requires an extra quarter mile of blood vessels, and his heart must beat harder and faster to supply this excess tissue with blood.

The term "overweight" is actually a misnomer. An obese person is really "overfat." A person can be carrying a lot of excess fat and not seem overweight at all. Take, for example, an ex-football player who has stayed the same weight as in his playing days but no longer exercises. His muscles in all likelihood have turned to fat.

The same thing happens to most adult Americans. During our teens, we are very active. But as we get into our late twenties, and even before, we start working at a steady, time-consuming job and we lose the desire, the time, and the inclination to exercise. Our bodies naturally turn soft.

The change doesn't happen all at once. But by the time we notice

25

IF FAT IS THE KILLER OF
THE HEART, WHY DON'T I
JUST GO ON A DIET?

the fat depositing around our middle, the degeneration of our muscles into fat has been going on for years. That's because it takes time for the subcutaneous fat to be deposited under the skin, and fat tissue weighs less than muscle tissue. You may weigh the same as you did in college, yet you probably have more fat now.

The standard height-weight charts simply are not geared to tell you whether you're "overfat." The only truly accurate gauge of how fat you are is your "lean body mass." Your lean body mass is the bone and muscle tissue of your body. If you subtract this mass from your actual gross weight, you can calculate how much of your weight is fat —in other words, your body-fat ratio.

The chart below indicates the body-fat ratio of men ranging from a very lean, highly trained athlete such as a long-distance runner to a very fat, sedentary man. Most of our adult population falls into the "overfat" or "obese" categories.

BODY-FAT RATIOS FOR MEN

Very Lean	8–10%
Lean	11–14%
Average	15–20%
Overfat	21–24%
Obese	25–28%

As noted earlier, the ideal body-fat ratio for adult men is 15 percent or below.

Tests to Determine Your Body-Fat Ratio

If you want to know if you're fat, a good way to test yourself is simply to stand in front of a full-length mirror without your clothes on. How do you look? Are you sagging where you never sagged before? Then you're probably fat.

Now give yourself the "pinch test." Take a fold of skin on the back of your upper arm between your thumb and forefinger. If you can pinch more than an inch of fat, you're probably not just fat but obese.

The pinched fat is subcutaneous fat—the fat lying directly beneath the skin—and this layer is consistent throughout your body. An inch of pinched fat usually means a body-fat ratio of around 30 percent.

An accurate skin-fold measurement can be taken with calipers specially calibrated for this purpose. For home use, a pair of plastic calipers, along with a chart of skin-fold thicknesses and your body-fat composition, can be obtained from Dr. H. Company, P.O. Box 266, Chesterfield, MO 63017 for $5.95 plus 50 cent handling. More accurate medical and research calipers can be purchased from medical supply stores, but they are more expensive.

Hydrostatic Weighing

By far, the most accurate method of determining your body-fat ratio is hydrostatic weighing. To do this, a person must be completely submerged in a tub of water; the amount of water he displaces is then measured. Other methods of determining body-fat ratio, such as skin-fold measurements, are not as accurate as hydrostatic weighing because they measure only subcutaneous fat. Hydrostatic weighing measures intramuscular fat as well and, therefore, can reveal how fat you truly are—even before it begins to show.

Unfortunately, hydrostatic weighing takes equipment that is both elaborate and expensive and, therefore, must be done at a professional clinic or medical facility. But it is well worth the time, trouble, and expense, if you want to find out how fat you really are.

Lack of Muscular Fitness Is the Problem— Not Overweight

Exercise, not diet, is the key to losing weight and keeping it off. When you exercise you not only lose weight—you lose fat. A person who undergoes a rapid weight loss on a diet often looks haggard and worn, and his skin looks as if it is just hanging on him. That is because dieting can lead to muscle deterioration. The weight you lose on a diet is due more to water loss than to fat loss. Dieting doesn't remove intramuscular fat and it's this fatty muscle tissue in your body that's the real problem. If you exercise while you diet, your muscles will remain firm and you will look better and feel better as you lose weight.

There are skeptics who will tell you that you can't burn up enough calories while exercising to make any difference in your weight. They like to bring up statistics; for instance, it takes almost forty miles of brisk walking to burn up one pound of fat, or if you jog for twenty minutes you'll burn up 180 calories, which you'll gain right back by drinking a glass of milk. These figures may be true technically, but the human body is too complex for mere statistics to tell the whole story. The "balance sheet" theory of weight loss—you put in so much food fuel and you do so much exercise and whatever is not used up is deposited as fat—is a myth because it completely ignores the *cumulative* effect of exercise.

27

IF FAT IS THE KILLER OF THE HEART, WHY DON'T I JUST GO ON A DIET?

Exercise changes your body chemistry and makes you a more efficient machine. The man who exercises burns his fuel differently than the sedentary man. Aerobic exercise raises your metabolic rate, so you're burning more calories, not only while engaging in vigorous exercise, but for hours afterward.

Also, physically fit people have a slightly higher body temperature due to their elevated metabolism. This causes them to burn calories at a faster rate even while they're sleeping.

Exercise, not diet, is the cure for a weight problem. The reason a person has trouble keeping weight off after a diet is because he has not changed his body chemistry. He is still fat. It's just a matter of time before his intramuscular fat turns to subcutaneous fat and that spare tire starts coming back.

Steady, continuous exercise is the best way to get fat off and keep it off, because aerobic exercise replaces fatty tissue with lean muscle tissue. Stop-and-start exercises, which use quick bursts of energy, burn pure glucose. And the body never gets a chance to tap its resources of fat.

There Is No Such Thing as Spot Reducing

Many people ask how to reduce weight around the midsection. The standard answer is situps. But the fat around your stomach, your "spare tire," belongs to your entire body. By overworking the muscles of your stomach, all you're doing is building a strong stomach. There is no such thing as spot reducing.

Calisthenics and weight lifting are fine for building up weak muscles, but they will not remove fat from a particular part of the body. One muscle or set of muscles exercised at a time simply cannot burn as much fat as many muscles working at once. You *can* get rid of intramuscular fat by exercising only that particular muscle or set of muscles. But a selective exercise such as situps will not eliminate subcutaneous fat in the area on *top* of that muscle. To eliminate fatty bulges on your body, particularly the stomach, you've got to do large muscle exercises, such as those described in this book.

It's clear that exercise—no matter what kind—reduces fat from all over the body and not from any specific area. And aerobic exercise is the most efficient exercise for burning fat. So if you want to lose that big stomach, if you want to rid your entire body of the fat that is choking the life and energy right out of you, you must put yourself on a regular program of aerobic exercise.

PART THREE

GETTING READY TO
GET FIT

CHAPTER 7

FINDING OUT HOW YOU TICK

The Heart Rate Is the True Measure of Exercise

The key to a successful aerobic exercise program is to make sure you don't exercise too much or too little. And to determine how much exercise is just right for you, you must have physical and numerical guidelines that are easy to follow. The ideal program must have an indicator of stress built into it, so each person can determine for himself when he has reached his limit.

In order to improve your condition and stamina, you must exercise so that you "overload" the body. In other words, you must expend more energy than you normally do. And you can do this by either exercising harder or longer than usual.

It stands to reason that the better shape you're in, the more strenuous your fitness routine must be to maintain your level of conditioning. If you haven't exercised in years, it's not going to take more than a walk around the block to get you in a little better shape tomorrow than you are in today. But that same walk wouldn't do a thing for a well-conditioned athlete.

It all gets down to how much effort each individual puts into an exercise. A man with well-developed muscles can lift five-pound weights most of the night and it won't improve his strength. But a weak, flabby man can build muscle tissue by leaps with the same exercise.

The old method of exercising, especially with calisthenics or weights, emphasized "fitness by the numbers." "Do twenty pushups, fifty situps, and run a mile . . ." But what if you're not as fit as the next guy, or you're in great shape but you've been sick for a while, or you're having an off day either physically or psychologically, or you're just not as young as you used to be? The numbers approach to exercise measures how much work you put in, but not how much effort. An easy workout will not do you as much good as one that takes a good deal of effort; but a program that's too tough—that you either can't finish or leaves you lame for a week—is not right for you either.

What we need is an exercise computer that can be hooked up to each person as he exercises. Then, when he's had just the right amount of exercise for that particular day, he can call it quits.

And in fact we have such a computer. *It's the heart.* How fast your heart is beating (your pulse rate) during exercise can be used to build an exercise program that fits your individual requirements. Your pulse rate is your guide to fitness.

There is a point during exercise at which you reach your maximum oxygen intake—when your heart and lungs cannot pump any more oxygen to your tissues. At this point, the oxygen being brought in by the lungs can't be delivered to the muscles fast enough to supply the energy needed for further exercise. In other words, you run out of gas.

When the body cannot supply any more oxygen, the heart will be unable to beat any faster. If you know what your maximum heart rate is, you can then gauge how much effort you are putting into your exercise simply by taking your pulse.

When you approach your maximum heart rate, you know you're overdoing it. But the next question is, how much is enough? Studies have shown that for the greatest improvement in your fitness the heart should be stressed at about 80 percent of its maximum.

As an exercise gauge, the heart is nearly infallible. If you can perform an exercise with ease, your heart rate remains low. If you're working hard, so is your heart. As you pick up the pace of your exercise, and exert yourself more and more, your heart beat rises accordingly.

But your heart rate is an indicator of many even more subtle variables—age, physical condition, sickness, depression, stress, and even atmospheric conditions such as a very hot, humid day or a very cold day.

Take, for example, those days when you're not feeling well. Maybe you're getting a cold, or you're just getting over the flu. You may feel well enough to exercise, but too much exercise, such as your regular workout, would probably send you back to bed again. On those days it takes less exercise, less exertion, to raise your heart level to about 80 percent of its maximum. If you're fatigued, you have to put out less effort to reach that training heart rate. By maintaining a constant heart rate while you exercise, you can maintain a constant level of effort.

Any change at all in your physical condition automatically is considered in determining how much you should exercise that day. When you're sick, your pulse rate responds more quickly to exertion and stress. The stronger you are, the more effort it will take to get your heart rate up.

The heart, therefore, is the universal measuring device for physical fitness.

Your Resting Heart Rate

While you are completely at rest your heart rate tells you a lot about your health and fitness. A man's normal resting heart rate averages between seventy-two and seventy-six beats per minute. But rates as low as forty and as high as ninety or a hundred can still be considered normal. For instance, many highly conditioned athletes, such as marathoners, have resting heart rates below forty.

In general, the lower your resting heart rate is, the healthier you are. For example, men with resting heart rates over ninety are four times more likely to have heart attacks than men with resting heart rates below seventy-two. A high resting heart rate is not a sure sign of poor health, but it does mean that the heart is working hard.

Your pulse rate during moderate exercise will rise to around 120 no matter what your resting heart rate is. So if your resting heart rate is over 100 while you're lying in bed, your heart is working almost as hard as that of someone moving at a brisk walk. And that's an unnecessary strain on your heart. A high resting rate is inefficient and exhausting for your whole system.

A lower rate, on the other hand, indicates that the heart is resting longer between beats and is pumping more efficiently. The blood flow is increased and so is the oxygen supply to the heart.

One important goal of a good fitness program should be to lower your resting heart rate. And the best way to do that is to make your heart beat faster for extended periods of time—in other words, by exercising aerobically.

How to Determine Your Resting Heart Rate

To determine your resting heart rate, sit quietly for thirty seconds, then take your pulse for thirty seconds and double the count. Take your pulse several times during the day to get an accurate measurement of your average resting heart rate.

How to Determine Your Maximum Heart Rate

Computing your maximum heart rate is really quite simple, because the only thing that affects it is age. The older you are, the slower your heart beats at its maximum. The most your heart will beat is about 220 times per minute, minus your age. In other words, if you're twenty, your maximum heart rate is around 200. For a forty-year-old, it's 180, and so on. The maximum heart rate, then, is the fastest your heart will beat for your age. (Do not exercise at this rate because it puts your heart at peak stress and you'll run out of gas long before you begin to burn fat or tone your muscles.)

Once again, the formula to determine your maximum heart rate is:

220 minus your age = maximum heart rate

How to Determine Your Training Heart Rate

Most normal, healthy individuals who want to benefit from aerobic exercise should exercise at a pace strenuous enough to raise their pulse rates to 80 percent of their maximum heart rate. This is your training heart rate.

The formula for determining your training heart rate is:

maximum heart rate $\times$ .80 = training heart rate

The heart rate during the first ten seconds after a strenuous workout is almost identical to the heart rate during peak exercise and, therefore, can accurately be used to determine your training heart rate. It is not necessary to take your pulse while you exercise!

AGE	HEART RATE	AGE	HEART RATE	AGE	HEART RATE
30	152	40	144	50	136
31	151	41	143	51	135
32	150	42	142	52	134
33	150	43	142	53	134
34	149	44	141	54	133
35	148	45	140	55	132
36	147	46	139	56	131
37	146	47	138	57	130
38	146	48	138	58	130
39	145	49	137	59	129
				60	128

Check your pulse immediately after you stop exercising. If your heart rate is ten beats slower than your calculated training heart rate, then you're not exercising hard enough. If your heart is beating ten beats faster than your training heart rate, you should exercise more slowly.

How to Determine Your Training Heart Rate if Your Resting Heart Rate Is Abnormally Low

The table for training heart rates (above) assumes that your resting heart beat is somewhere near the average for men—about seventy-two beats per minute. If, however, your resting heart rate is abnormally low, say in the forty-to-fifty-beats-per-minute range, then it will take a great deal of exertion to push your heart rate as high as a person's whose resting heart rate is much faster. So, for those of you with resting heart rates fifteen beats or more below average, it's probably safer to use the following formula when calculating your training heart rate.

(maximum heart rate − resting heart rate) × .65 + resting heart rate = training heart rate

For example, if you are a forty-year-old man whose resting heart rate is fifty, then your training heart rate is 134.

Heart Recovery Rate

Another reliable indicator of your fitness is your heart recovery rate. When you stop exercising, your heart beat begins to return quickly to its resting heart rate. The speed with which the heart recovers reflects the efficiency of your cardiovascular system. This slowdown of the heart follows two stages. First, immediately after you stop exercising, the pulse drops sharply for a while and levels off. Then, your pulse gradually decreases until your heart is beating at its original resting rate.

The heart may stay at the rate at which it leveled off for quite some time before it goes all the way back down to the resting heart rate. But this is insignificant. It's only your heart rate at the first plateau that matters. A healthy heart recovers more quickly than one not used to a strenuous workout.

Here's how to determine your heart recovery rate: after you exercise vigorously for a few minutes, raising your heart rate to your training rate, stop and rest for sixty seconds. Now count your pulse for thirty seconds. If you count more than sixty-five beats (130 per minute), you're probably out of shape.

When you're fit, your heart will probably beat about fifty times every half minute at the first plateau, no matter how hard you exercise.

How to Take Your Pulse

In order to ensure that you're maintaining a training-level heart rate and thereby engaging in aerobic exercise, you need to know how to take your pulse.

There are two very simple ways to check your pulse. The first is to place your middle fingers over one of the carotid arteries beneath your jaw on either side of your neck. *Warning:* don't press too hard; it could cause the heart to slow by reflex. The second method is to turn one hand palm up and place the middle three fingers of the other hand on the thumb side of your wrist; move them around until you feel your blood pulsing. Don't take your pulse with your thumb because it has a pulse of its own; if you feel two pulses you'll become confused when you try to count.

Once you have found your pulse either at the carotid artery of the neck or the radial artery of your wrist, count the pulse beats for six

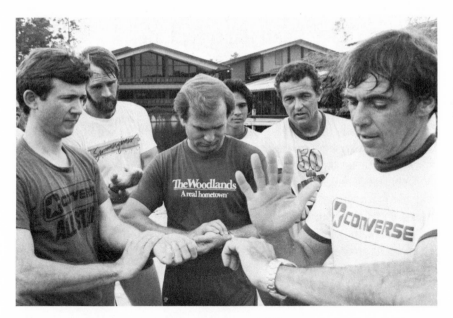

To take your pulse, place your middle fingers on either the carotid artery of the neck or the radial artery of the wrist, as shown. Count your pulse for six seconds and multiply by ten.

seconds and multiply this number by ten. This will give you the amount of beats per minute.

Even though you can get a more accurate pulse by taking a longer count, say for thirty seconds or a full minute, this will not reflect your pulse rate while exercising. The heart rate decreases rapidly as soon as you stop exercising, and after thirty seconds the difference can be as much as thirty beats from your training heart rate.

Practice the six-second pulse count so you can take your pulse rapidly. You'll have a fast, efficient, and accurate method of determining your training heart rate. And you'll know if the exercise you're doing is intense enough to improve your cardiovascular fitness.

As you grow fitter, your pulse will feel more forceful because your heart is getting stronger and your arteries are expanding to accommodate the greater volume of blood flowing through your veins. Also, as the weeks pass, your pulse rate will be lower after exercise of the same intensity.

The Intensity, Duration, and Frequency of Your Workout

For an aerobic exercise program to get you fit, three factors are essential: first, the exercise must be intense enough; second, it must be done without interruption for a sufficient period of time; and, third, you must repeat the exercise often enough. Once a month won't do anything but give you sore muscles every thirty days.

How much, how long, and how frequent should your aerobic exercise program be?

How Hard Should I Exercise?

The intensity of the exercise program depends completely on the individual. Two people can exercise exactly the same amount for the same length of time, and when they're through, one might not even be breathing hard and the other might not be breathing at all. Too much or too little exercise won't get you in shape. Unfortunately, most exercise programs either start you out too quickly or too slowly.

That's why a heart-regulated exercise program is ideal. No matter how out of shape you are, you only need put enough exertion into your exercise to lift your pulse to your ideal training rate. The heart rate is easy to check and it is totally relative to you and your physical condition.

If your pulse rate is within ten beats of your training range, you're exercising at the right rate. If it's lower than the training rate, you're exercising too lightly and you should pick up the pace. Check your pulse often. You'll probably find that after a few days the same amount of exercise won't tire you as much. Your heart will tell you when to step up your exercise.

If your heart rate is higher than your training rate should be, if it is, in fact, climbing close to your maximum heart rate—slow down! Remember, aerobic exercise is meant to make your muscles work hard enough to demand plenty of oxygen but not so hard that your cardiovascular and respiratory systems can't meet that demand.

Do not exceed your training heart rate! The muscles should be working only hard enough to bring in oxygen at a steady but vigorous rate. You should not be in pain or struggling to keep up. The old adage "the more it hurts, the better it is for you" is wrong. If your exercise is so intense that it hurts, your muscles are fatiguing. Lactic acid is building up in your muscles, causing pain and, eventually, muscle failure. That won't do you any good—and it could hurt you.

How Long and How Often Should I Exercise?

It's been found that following a fitness routine in which you exercise aerobically (with your heart rate at its training level) for at least twelve minutes will strengthen your heart and lungs, burn calories, eliminate body poisons, and keep you fit.

Why twelve minutes? Well, we don't know exactly. But we do know that if you bring your heart rate up to 80 percent of its maximum and keep it there for twelve minutes, you will have tapped into the fat supplies of your body and increased the capacities of your cardiovascular and respiratory systems.

The next question is: if I exercise for more than twelve minutes, will my fitness improve at a quicker rate? Yes, it will. But after the first twelve minutes, the same exercise is not as effective. Exercising for twenty-four minutes, three times a week, is not as effective as exercising for twelve minutes, six times a week.

I suggest a *minimum* workout of twenty minutes, including a warm-up, a twelve-minute aerobic workout, and a cool-down. Ideally, if you have the time, you should exercise for forty-five minutes, with twenty minutes devoted strictly to aerobics. But if you only have the time for the twenty-minute program, then that is certainly adequate to improve and maintain your cardiovascular fitness.

How often should you exercise? Studies have shown that the body begins to lose its conditioning seventy-two hours after exercising. Therefore, an exercise program will be less effective if there are more than two days between sessions. Most find that an every-other-day schedule for cardiovascular training is the minimum necessary to keep fit. You should exercise at least three or four times a week, five if you're looking for ideal results. Researchers at the Western Psychiatric Institute in Pittsburgh, for example, found that people who exercised five times a week lost half a pound of fat a week—three times more than those people who exercised only three times a week.

But don't overdo it. More than five times a week doesn't provide enough rest for the muscles to recuperate and grow. If you exercise too often, you won't recover totally between workouts and fatigue will prevent you from maintaining the intensity level best suited for you.

I suggest you follow the exercise schedule that fits you best. Ideally, a forty-five-minute program performed four or five times a week will bring you the fastest and the best results. If you're pressed for time, follow the twenty-minute program every day, if possible, but at least three times a week; you will steadily improve your health. Perhaps, as you feel better, you'll find more time. It's amazing how much energy you have when you're fit. One of the first things people who begin an exercise program report is that they need less sleep. After following the twenty-minute program for a while, you'll soon have the extra twenty-five minutes you need to follow the forty-five-minute workout.

CHAPTER 8

HOW FIT ARE YOU? EVALUATING YOUR PHYSICAL FITNESS

If You Have Any Doubt, Get a Physical

Before you begin a serious exercise program, you should know just how fit you are. Normally, if you're under thirty years old and have had no serious medical problems, a sensible workout should be completely safe. But even under those ideal circumstances, you should have a physical examination by a doctor before you undertake a strenuous exercise program.

Most Americans—especially men—feel that they are in better shape than they are. They attack an exercise program as vigorously as they played sports in high school. They're competitive; they want to win everything they get involved in—even if it's jogging. If you're like me, you'll go out there and try to beat your buddy George around that track. If George can do eight laps, you can do ten—even if it kills you.

This competitive drive is admirable, but it can also be dangerous. An unconditioned body that has had little or no regular exercise for ten, twenty, or even thirty years is prone to serious injury and possibly fatal coronary complications. Therefore, I urge you to heed these words: unless you have had one recently, get a thorough physical examination *before* you start exercising in earnest.

Any physical examination you have should include a complete medical history and a thorough testing of the cardiovascular system, including heart rate, blood pressure, and blood analysis with emphasis on cholesterol, triglycerides, and a blood count. Also, an electrocardiogram should be taken while you're at rest and while you're exercising, if possible. In addition, make sure that a chest X-ray, urinalysis, and examination of the muscles and joints is included.

After your physical—unless your doctor specifically recommends against it—you should be able to begin your aerobic workout. But let me warn you, if you have any of the following problems, exercise only under the strictest of medical supervision:

coronary or valvular heart disease
diabetes
liver problems, especially accompanied by jaundice
hemorrhaging
high blood pressure
high cholesterol
a history of family heart disease
dizziness or fainting
pains in the chest
difficulty in breathing
heavy smoking
tendon or cartilage injuries affecting movement
recent surgery
a recent serious illness

Fitness Tests You Can Perform Yourself

There are some simple yet relatively accurate methods of testing your own physical fitness. The tests listed below will give you a clear idea of how your physical condition measures up in the five important categories of fitness: cardiovascular fitness, body-fat ratio, flexibility, muscular strength, and muscular endurance. (The body-fat ratio tests —the pinch test and hydrostatic weighing—have already been described in Chapter 6.)

The Step Test

This is a very effective and informative test, yet one that is simple to take at home. It's safe enough to be taken by most people, except the sick or extremely obese or unfit. However, if easy exercise such as walking up a flight of stairs leaves you breathless, don't attempt any unsupervised testing. Also, stop any test or exercise if you experience such symptoms of heart trouble as dizziness, pain or tightness in the chest, severe shortness of breath, or nausea.

To administer this self-test, you need a bench or step exactly twelve inches high and a watch with a sweep hand.

Step up and down from the bench for three minutes at a rate of twenty-four per minute. Both feet must step onto the bench and return to the floor each time in a four-count rhythm: 1) step up with the right foot; 2) step up with the left foot; 3) step down with the right; 4) step down with the left. Rehearse this rhythm, up and down once every two and a half seconds, before you start the test. Try to keep a relaxed even motion. Don't jump up to the bench. Also, extend the legs fully on each step.

At the end of three minutes, sit down and relax completely for five seconds. Now take your pulse for a full sixty seconds and compare your results with the norms for young and middle-aged men listed below.

CONDITION	PULSE RATE: AGE 20–35	PULSE RATE: AGE 35–55
Excellent	69–75	75–80
Good	76–85	85–90
Average	86–92	95–115
Fair	93–99	120–125
Poor	100–106	130–135

The fitter you are, the less the pulse rate rises initially and the faster the pulse rate recovers. A lower total means higher cardiovascular fitness. This is not a substitute for a standard stress test, but it can tell you a lot about your aerobic capacity and your ability to undertake a strenuous aerobic workout.

A Simple Flexibility Test

It's difficult to get an accurate measurement of flexibility by a simple test because this often varies from joint to joint. You may have the total range of movement in your right shoulder and almost none in your right knee. However, the elasticity of the lower back, the thighs, and the hamstrings have been found to be a relatively reliable indicator of an individual's overall flexibility. The sitting toe touch involves these muscles and, therefore, can give you a fairly good idea of your flexibility.

In order to avoid injury during this test, do a few warm-up stretches first. Rotate the trunk slowly and without jerky movements.

1. Put a strip of adhesive tape about two feet long onto the floor. Have a yardstick ready.
2. Sit on the floor with your feet facing the strip of adhesive and extend your legs fully, with the heels approximately six inches apart and just touching the tape.

3. Place the yardstick on the floor between your legs so that the fifteen-inch mark is at the edge of the tape where your heels are. (Be sure that inches one through fifteen of the yardstick are between your legs and inches fifteen through thirty-six are beyond the tape line.)
4. Slowly stretch both hands as far forward as possible and place your fingertips on the yardstick. Hold this position for a moment. Note the distance you've reached on the yardstick. Don't try for more length by rocking forward!
5. Try this three times. Your best score is your flexibility rating.

FLEXIBILITY RATINGS

22–23 inches	Excellent
20–21	Good
14–19	Average
12–13	Fair
0–11	Poor

The Grip-Strength Test

As with flexibility, measuring overall muscular strength is not easy because there are so many different muscles and muscle groups. But we can measure the strength of one muscle group that most closely correlates with the body's overall muscular strength.

The grip-strength test is used most often to determine overall strength. You need a hand-grip dynamometer for this test. Squeeze the dynamometer as hard as possible with your dominant hand. The device measures resistance, which reflects your relative strength. The drawback to this test, of course, is that you've got to find a dynamometer. The dynamometer can be bought from medical supply stores, one of which is Livingstone Home Care, 628 Ocean Street, Santa Cruz, California, 95060. The price is approximately $170.00 and your inquiry should be addressed care of Bruce Rowe.

Minimum-Strength Test

An even simpler way to measure your strength is the minimum-strength test, developed by Dr. Hans Kraus. You can only pass or fail this series of tests. If you fail any of them, your body is seriously under strength in the area tested, and this weakness could affect the health of your entire body.

1. Lie on your back with your hands behind your neck. Have someone hold your feet down and then do one situp. This tests your stomach and loin muscles.

2. Start in the same position as test number 1. Then bend your knees and move your heels up close to your buttocks. Do one situp. This tests your stomach muscles, unaided by your loin muscles.
3. Start in the same position as number 1. Then lift your legs, fully extended, until your heels are about twelve inches off the ground. Hold that position for ten seconds. This tests your lower stomach and loin muscles.
4. Lie face down with a pillow under your hips and stomach. Put your hands behind your neck and have someone hold your feet down. Raise your head, shoulders, and chest and hold them off the floor for ten seconds. This tests your upper-back muscles.
5. Start in the same position as number 4. Have someone hold your shoulders down. Raise your legs off the floor, keeping your knees straight. Hold that position for ten seconds. This tests the strength of your lower back.
6. Do one pushup. (Lie face down on the floor with your feet together and your palms on the floor next to your shoulders. Keeping your body straight, push yourself off the floor by straightening your arms.)

Muscular-Endurance Test

Because it involves one of the body's most important muscle groups, the situp is a fairly reliable indicator of muscular endurance.

Lie flat on your back on the floor with your knees bent and the soles of your feet flat on the floor. Put your hands behind your head and have someone hold your feet down. Now lift your trunk up and touch your right elbow to your left knee, and go back down again. Then lift up and touch your left elbow to your right knee. Do as many situps as you can without stopping, being sure to breathe freely. Then count your total and look at the chart below to find out how fit you are.

MUSCULAR ENDURANCE RATINGS

NUMBER OF SITUPS	ENDURANCE
less than 15	Poor
15–34	Fair
35–59	Average
60–100	Good
over 100	Superior

The purpose of all these tests is simply to put your individual fitness in perspective. You can find out through your scores how you compare to other people. Remember, however, that these tests are not meant to be competitive. So don't strain yourself trying to outperform a friend. Properly used, these tests can give you a clear indication of where you need improvement and which exercises you should concentrate on in your workout.

PART FOUR

THE AEROBIC WORKOUT
FOR MEN

CHAPTER 9

BEFORE YOU START

In order to enhance your understanding and enjoyment of the Aerobic Workout for Men, here are a few things to think about before you start your workout.

Start Easy—Progress Gradually

The two main questions I always hear from beginners are: "Where do I start?" and "How fast should I progress?"

Whether you've just turned thirty and are only beginning to turn to fat, or you're fifty and haven't seen your feet in years, the first principle of any sound fitness program is to slowly ease your way into it.

We've become an instant society. We've got instant coffee, overnight mail service, and ovens that can cook a meal in twenty minutes. Wherever we go we always seem to have to be there yesterday. But you can't rush things when it comes to conditioning your body. *There is no instant fitness.*

The importance of patience when exercising cannot be overemphasized. When I first started my own aerobic workout, my goal was to lose eighteen pounds. I sweated and strained for a week and a half and I lost exactly three-quarters of a pound. I was stiff all over and in pain when I walked. But I had the faith to stick with it. After the second week, I started to show real improvement. I dropped as much as a half a pound a day for weeks. The aches went away as quickly as they had come and I felt great.

You've got to have patience—and you've got to be realistic. It took you ten, twenty, thirty years to get out of shape, so it would be unreasonable to expect to get back in shape in a matter of days.

Most fitness experts agree that it takes anywhere from six to ten weeks to get a normal beginner into good enough shape to be ready for the challenges of true fitness.

Besides, there are strong risks involved in trying to do too much too soon—like trying to shed thirty pounds of fat and overcome thirty years of inactivity in thirty days. If you progress gradually, you will accustom the heart to the demands of aerobic exercise and avoid strains and pulls to muscles and tendons. And simple muscular soreness can be kept to a minimum that way.

Even if you're in shape for a sport such as tennis, racquetball, or jogging, you may not be in shape for aerobic exercises. So start in a beginner's class and stay there at least one week. If it's not strenuous enough, jump to a more advanced class the following week. But let me warn you: I have never seen anyone, not even a world-class athlete, join a good aerobics class and not find the beginner's workout extremely challenging for at least one or two weeks. After this breaking-in period, the better-conditioned athletes progress more rapidly than the unfit, but they still must go through this initial period to accustom themselves and their muscles to these new exercises.

If for any reason you stop doing your aerobic workout for more than two weeks, don't return to it at the same level as when you left. Significant conditioning is lost during any lay-off from exercise. This is particularly true if you were forced to stop exercising due to sickness, which tends to weaken the body in general.

The Age Factor

A man reaches his peak physical condition between twenty-five and thirty years of age. After that, his strength, speed, and reflexes slowly decline until age fifty, when they drop off even more rapidly. His maximum heart rate and oxygen intake follow a similar decline.

This means that an older man's physical condition will improve more slowly with exercise. Also, a man over thirty gets out of shape more quickly. As a result, the intensity, duration, and frequency of an older man's exercise will not be the same as when he was younger.

Because the efficiency of the heart, lungs, and muscles of even a healthy middle-aged man is lower than that of a young man, some restraint is required. With rare exception, an athlete is old by the time he's thirty-five. Still, no matter what age we are, many of us believe we're capable of doing exactly what we did ten years ago.

There's no doubt that a well-conditioned man of fifty can keep up with or even beat the average thirty-year-old. But you cannot make up for thirty years of neglect overnight.

You can still get a middle-aged body in shape, but it's going to take a little longer. You're going to have to spend a lot more time warming up your body before you exercise. Loosen up and get that warm, flushed feeling. And, by all means, listen to your body! If it tells you to stop—then stop! Your body will also signal when you're ready to exercise more vigorously.

Keep Moving

The most important thing to keep in mind while doing the aerobic exercise portion of the workout is that you must keep moving. You must keep your heart beating at its training rate to accomplish the physiological goals of an aerobics workout.

If you can't keep up with the group or you can't get your body to perform a certain exercise, then simply jog in place until it's time to move on to another exercise, or until you catch your breath. If you get bored with jogging, you can hop from one foot to another and wave your arms around in some rhythmic fashion. But keep moving!

Put Variety in Your Workout

The major drawback to most exercise programs is that the instructor stays far too long on each exercise. He pushes the participants through the workout, staying on each exercise "until it hurts." But aerobic exercise was designed specifically *not* to strain the muscles.

As you exercise, keep shifting the workload from one muscle group to another to avoid fatigue. Stay with one exercise no more than thirty seconds. Remember, as soon as you feel your muscles fatiguing, switch to another exercise.

Varying your exercises frequently throughout your workout also prevents boredom—a major enemy of a regular exercise routine.

Don't Exercise by the Numbers

Since arm strength may progress faster than, say, leg strength, or cardiovascular fitness faster than muscular fitness, only do each exercise as long as you can without straining excessively. Don't try to do fifty situps when you can only do thirty comfortably.

In other words, don't exercise by the numbers! That's the old method of exercising—with a drill instructor ordering you to "gut it out." This is a new, enlightened era of exercise. Just because you can do twenty situps, doesn't mean you can do twenty leg lifts.

Another thing. In the "Floor Exercises" section of the Advanced Workout, I suggest that you do a certain number of repetitions of each exercise. But the numbers should serve as a guide only. Do not overexercise!

Do Each Exercise Correctly

Most people think of exercise as movement. The more you move, the better. The higher you kick, the farther you stretch, the fitter you'll be. But often the effectiveness of an exercise comes from doing a little less, a little better. Do every exercise as correctly as you possibly can. Keep the right alignment. Breathe deeply. Exercise every muscle that's supposed to be exercised.

If an exercise hurts, stop. You may be doing it wrong, so check the instructions again. If it still hurts, have a friend watch you do the exercise, or check with an aerobics instructor.

Breathing Your Fat Away

As I've said before, getting oxygen into your body is the key to fitness. Breathing supplies oxygen to the muscles, heart, and lungs, which is what aerobic exercise is all about. The so-called "burning away of fat" depends on the oxygen intake capability of the person exercising. The bloodstream also carries away waste products and toxic gases—a lot of which are exhaled directly out through the lungs.

Therefore, it is important that you breathe deeply and regularly throughout your workout. Get that oxygen into your bloodstream. As your muscles demand more oxygen, the heart pumps faster and the lungs, in turn, must send larger amounts of oxygen into the bloodstream. So, as a general principle, you should breathe more deeply and more often as you exercise harder.

The Importance of the Music

Don't mistake the workout in this book for a dance class. The music, however, is very important to the enjoyment and effectiveness of the exercises. Playing music while you exercise helps you concentrate, keeps you going when you want to quit, and cuts boredom. It simply makes the time that you spend working and sweating a lot more enjoyable.

I have included a list of songs to go with each of the four sections of the workout: "The Warm-up," "The Aerobic Exercises," "The Floor Exercises," and "The Cool-down." Each section has a different intensity, rhythm, and mood and the music was selected with this in mind. But the songs listed are really only suggestions. I urge you to make up a tape of your own favorite tunes that have the right tempo and the right mood to help you exercise.

Slow, mellow music is probably best for "The Warm-up" and "The Cool-down," and upbeat music for "The Aerobic Exercises" and "The Floor Exercises." You've got to get your blood moving and "Moon River" just won't do it. If you're a little out of touch with the latest dance music, ask your kids to put together a tape for you. Show them a few exercises and they'll figure out what you need.

Also, record the songs on a ninety-minute, long-playing cassette. One side runs for forty-five minutes, so you can get through your entire workout without stopping to flip it over. When the cassette is through, so are you.

Once you've got your music, you're ready to start exercising. All you need is your cassette recorder and your music and you're all set to get in shape. Or, if you've left your tape at home, tune the radio to a station with upbeat music.

The Importance of the Warm-up and the Cool-down

Warming Up

Whether you're just beginning to exercise again after a long layoff or you're as fit as a marathoner, be sure to warm up before engaging in *any* exercise.

The warm-up is designed to get your body ready for vigorous exertion. It raises your heart rate toward the training rate, warms and stretches your muscles, and gets that stiff and lethargic feeling out of your body. A warmer body temperature increases the potential for greater movement, strength, and elasticity of tendons, ligaments, and muscles. It also reduces the risk of injury.

Stretching and Flexibility

Flexibility is the range of possible movement in a joint or series of joints. The need for flexibility varies with the activity or sport. But even for an armchair athlete, flexibility is important just to walk correctly. An improper gait caused by stiffness often results in lower-back problems. Maintaining flexibility often prevents or relieves the aches and pains that grow more common as you age and frequently precede arthritis.

Basically, there are three reasons we need to stretch our muscles: 1) to improve our range of motion, 2) to help relieve muscle soreness after overexertion, and 3) to help prevent injury.

There are two types of stretching exercises. Dynamic stretching requires bobbing, bouncing, and jerking movements to reach the desired stretch. Static stretching is a slow, sustained stretching of the muscles and tendons in which a static position is held for ten to twenty seconds.

Both methods satisfactorily stretch the muscles, but there are distinct advantages to static stretching. For example, there is less danger of overstretching muscle tissue. Remember, muscles are like rubber bands. If you continue to pull on a rubber band in quick, jerky motions, it probably will break (like tearing a muscle); but if you gradually stretch the rubber band, you will eventually feel the limit of its elasticity. In static stretching, this is where you hold the position. Also, dynamic stretching often causes muscle soreness, whereas static stretching can actually relieve it. I use only static stretching exercises in this book.

One thing to remember about stretching: men generally don't have the same degree of flexibility as women. So don't try to imitate your wife or girlfriend; you may not necessarily be able to touch your fingers to your toes or your palms to the floor. Because we all vary so drastically in our body types and the length of our body parts, there are no standards for ideal flexibility. It is only important that you are at least flexible enough to move efficiently and minimize the risk of injury.

Cooling Down

A proper cool-down after working out is extremely important. The cool-down allows your heart to slow down gradually and helps return the body to its normal temperature. It also relaxes the muscles after their strenuous activity and helps expel the toxic wastes that accumulate in the muscles after exercises. If you don't cool down properly, cramping, tightness, and soreness of the muscles may result.

Be sure to taper off gradually after any exercise. Don't just fall on the bed or slump in the nearest chair. Also, avoid jumping right into a hot shower immediately after exercising. At least wait until you've stopped sweating.

Also, during the cool-down, it's a good idea to slip on your warm-up pants if you worked out in shorts. Also, don't turn on the air conditioner or fan and don't open any windows if it's cold outside.

Which Workout Should You Choose: The Get-in-Shape and Maintenance Workout or The Advanced Workout or The Super Workout?

The Get-in-Shape and Maintenance Workout

I suggest that everyone who is not now regularly following an aerobics program start with the Get-in-Shape and Maintenance Workout. It is designed to get you ready for the Advanced Workout or to maintain your present level of cardiovascular fitness on the days when you just don't have the time to do the Advanced Workout.

The Get-in-Shape and Maintenance Workout takes only about twenty minutes to complete. It includes a five-minute warm-up, twelve minutes of aerobic exercises, and a three-minute cool-down.

The Advanced Workout

If you're in good shape already and you can complete the Get-in-Shape Workout without much strain, move on to the Advanced Workout. The Advanced Workout is a more intense, thorough, and longer workout designed to get you in top physical shape and keep you that way. It includes floor exercises to develop your muscular strength and endurance and help burn away intramuscular fat.

The Advanced Workout takes about forty-five minutes and includes a six- to eight-minute warm-up, twenty minutes of aerobic exercises, fifteen minutes of floor exercises, and a four- to six-minute cool-down.

The Super Workout for the Super Athlete

The Super Workout for the Super Athlete is a sports-conditioning program designed for the rigors of competition. It is based on the Advanced Workout, except that the recommended training heart rates are higher. Included are workout suggestions and tips to help you perform better. The Super Workout is designed for an athlete involved in high school, university, and professional competition.

How to Follow the Workout

All of the exercises in the workouts include a thorough, step-by-step explanation of each exercise, with accompanying photos. So there's no guesswork. But in the beginning, you'll have to refer back and forth to the text and that may slow you down as you exercise. It's best to study the workout you're going to do beforehand. Read it through several times and rehearse a few of the more difficult exercises to see if you've got them right. Eventually, you should know the whole routine by heart, so you can go through it without stopping. Remember, you want to keep moving in order to keep your heart rate up. Finally, the exercises have been arranged in a sequence that is easy to follow. So do them in order.

Now, all that's left for you to do is face the music. And enjoy yourself.

CHAPTER 10

THE GET-IN-SHAPE AND MAINTENANCE WORKOUT

The Get-in-Shape and Maintenance Workout is designed to get you ready for the Advanced Workout. If you are already in shape, it will maintain your cardiovascular fitness on the days when you just don't have the time to do the Advanced Workout.

LENGTH OF WORKOUT: 20 minutes
FREQUENCY: at least 3 or 4 times a week, daily if possible

The Get-in-Shape and Maintenance Warm-up

5 MINUTES

The warm-up exercises loosen the muscles, warm the body, and prepare the cardiovascular system for the strenuous exercise to come. They also reduce the risk of injury.

☐ If you don't have an exercise mat, lay a large towel or blanket on the floor, preferably carpeted, so you have a clean, comfortable place to exercise.

☐ Only stretch as far as you can comfortably reach. *Do not bounce* to increase your reach. Feel the stretch and then hold the position for ten to twenty seconds.

☐ Breathe normally and regularly throughout the stretches.

☐ Go through all the stretches, and if you still don't feel warm and limber, go through them once again.

Suggested Music

SONG TITLE	ARTIST	ALBUM TITLE
"Blue Bayou"	Linda Ronstadt	*Simple Dreams*
"Design for Living"	Nona Hendryx	*Nona Hendryx*
"Georgia"	Boz Scaggs	*Silk Degrees*
"Fairy Tale High"	Donna Summer	*Live and More*
"Keep It Confidential"	Nona Hendryx	*Nona Hendryx*
"Mexico"	James Taylor	*James Taylor's Greatest Hits*

Exercise #1 Side Bends

Clasping your arms over your head, feet shoulder width apart, bend sideways at the waist as far as you can to the left, making sure you don't turn the upper torso. Keep the stomach and buttocks pulled in and bend straight to the side, then do the same exercise to the right. This is only beneficial if you stretch as far as possible. You may also rotate slowly in a circle, keeping your legs and hips in place. If you are particularly stiff, you can do Single Side Bends. Simply stretch one arm over your head while placing the other arm on your hip.

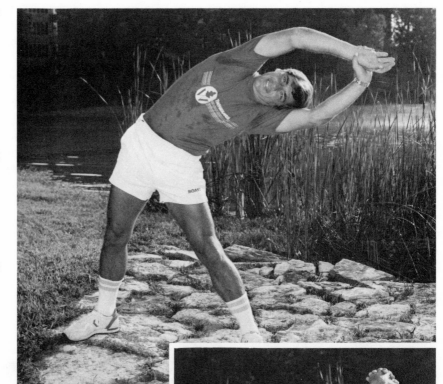

Exercise #2
Overhead Arm Stretch

With your feet about two inches apart and your legs straight, clasp your hands behind your back and bring them up as you bend forward at the waist. As your chest and arm muscles stretch out, bend a little farther forward. Do not strain.

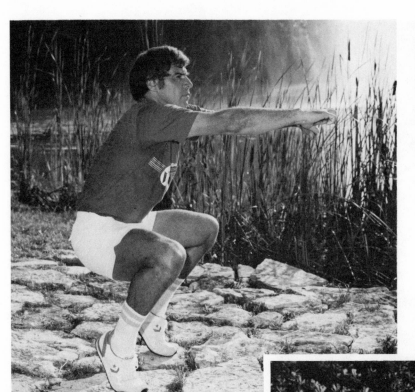

Exercise #3
Knee Bends
With your arms straight out in front of you, squat down, keeping your back straight. Raise up on your toes and hold for a few seconds. Do not let your buttocks go any lower than the level of your knees. Deep knee bends can be dangerous.

Exercise #4   Crossovers
Bending forward at the waist, try to touch your hands to the ground. Do not strain or bounce. Keeping your legs straight, cross your left foot over your right foot. Hold for a few seconds, return to a position with your feet together, and then cross your right foot over your left foot and stretch again. A lot of runners use Crossovers to stretch their hamstrings.

Exercise #5
Skier's Stretch
With your feet a little farther apart than shoulder width and your knees bent, turn your ankles out slowly and push out on your knees. This is an excellent exercise for tennis players, skiers, hockey players, or anyone involved in a sport that fosters frequent ankle injuries.

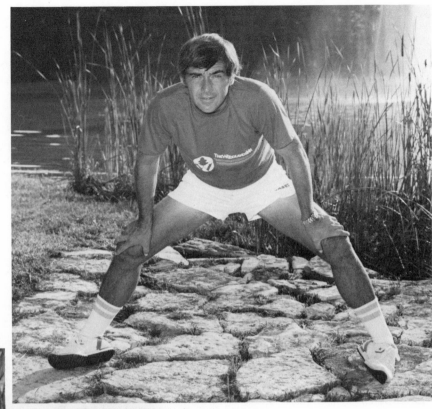

Exercise #6
Hand Walks
With your feet as wide apart as possible, walk your hands back between your legs as far as you can. Do not strain.
   Keep breathing normally! Do not hold your breath.

61

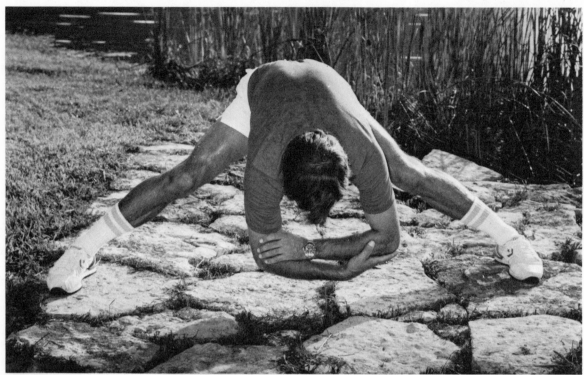

Exercise #7
Back Stretch

With your feet as wide apart as possible, cross your arms. Bending at the waist, try to touch your arms to the ground. Do not bounce! It is important to keep the legs straight.

Exercise #8
Runner's Stretch

With both heels flat on the ground and your legs straight, walk your hands forward as far as you can without bringing your heels off the ground.

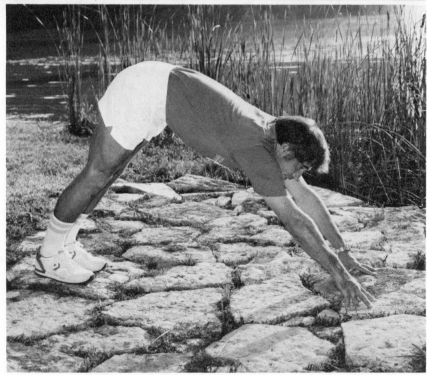

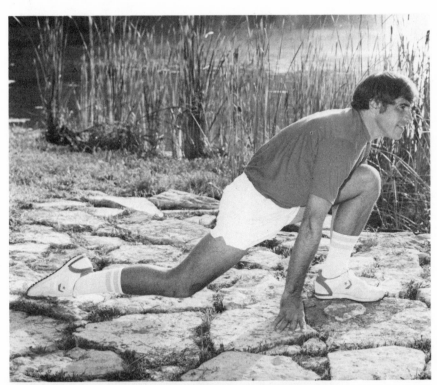

Exercise #9
Hurdler's Stretch
Position your left leg forward and your right leg behind. (Make sure that the top of the foot is on the ground as in the photograph.) Keep your left heel on the ground and feel the stretch in the back of your right thigh. Switch the position of your legs to stretch the left leg.

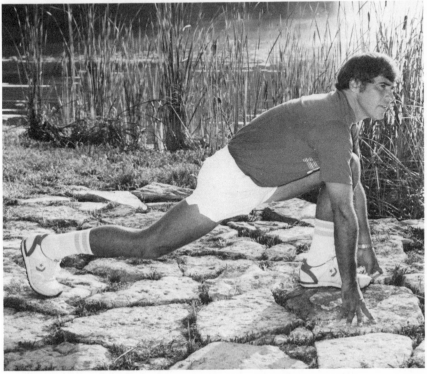

Exercise #10
Modified Hurdler's Stretch
From the position in figure 13, transfer the weight to the toes of the right leg by rocking back slowly and gently. Make sure that the left heel remains on the ground.

THE GET-IN-SHAPE AND MAINTENANCE WORKOUT

The Get-in-Shape and Maintenance Aerobic Exercises

12 MINUTES

The aerobic exercises are designed to build your cardiovascular fitness.

☐ In order to improve your cardiovascular fitness, you must keep moving throughout the aerobic exercises, so that your heart will continue to beat at your training rate.

☐ If the workout seems too strenuous for you, do the aerobic exercises to a little slower music. Or, when you get tired and winded, you can jog in place or do the "resting kick" (shown in figure 15) between exercises until you can get through the entire workout. You can also make the exercises easier by not using your arms. Rest your hands on your hips while you exercise.

☐ To make the exercises *more* strenuous, simply exaggerate all the movements of the arms and legs. Punch your fists out and then up. Kick your legs higher.

☐ Do each exercise for no more than thirty seconds. Then move on to the next exercise. As soon as you feel your muscles fatiguing, switch to another exercise.

☐ *Do not hold your breath.* It is important that you breathe deeply and regularly throughout the workout, but especially during the aerobic exercises.

☐ To ensure that you're exercising at your proper training rate throughout the aerobic exercises, take your pulse twice during this part of the workout.

Suggested Music

SONG TITLE	ARTIST	ALBUM TITLE
"The Eye of the Tiger"	Survivor	*The Eye of the Tiger*
"Walk Right Now"	The Jacksons	*Triumph*
"Gloria"	Laura Branigan	*Branigan*
"Abracadabra"	The Steve Miller Band	*Abracadabra*
"Hungry Like the Wolf"	Duran Duran	*Rio*
"Overkill"	Men at Work	*Cargo*
"One Thing Leads to Another"	The Fixx	*Reach the Beach*
"Baby Jane"	Rod Stewart	*Body Wishes*

"Physical"	Olivia Newton-John	*Physical*
"We Got the Beat"	The Go Go's	*Beauty and the Beat*
"You Should Be Dancing"	The Bee Gee's	*Bee Gee's Greatest Hits*
"We Made It"	Toto	*Toto IV*
"What a Feeling"	Irene Cara	*Flashdance*
"Space Age Love"	A Flock of Seagulls	*A Flock of Seagulls*
"Bad Girls"	Donna Summer	*Bad Girls*
"She Works Hard for the Money"	Donna Summer	*She Works Hard for the Money*
"Beat It"	Michael Jackson	*Thriller*
"Billie Jean"	Michael Jackson	*Thriller*
"P.Y.T."	Michael Jackson	*Thriller*

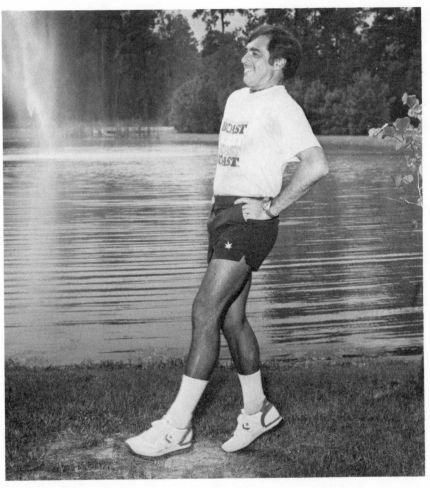

Exercise #1
Resting Kick
With your hands on your hips, lean slightly back and jump steadily on one leg and kick with the other. Alternate legs every two jumps.
Note: If you get too tired to continue the workout, use the Resting Kick or simply jog in place to catch your breath, then continue the workout. To vary this exercise you can also use arm movements, such as boxer's punches, while you do the kick.

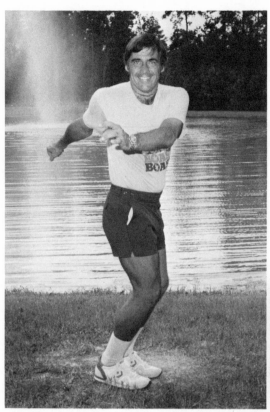

Exercise #2
Jump and Twist
Twist from side to side on both feet while swinging the arms to the opposite side of the body.

Exercise #3
Skipping Rope
This exercise is just like skipping rope, but without the rope. There are innumerable variations of this aerobic movement (for example, hopping twice on one foot and alternating to the other foot, keeping the movement continuous).

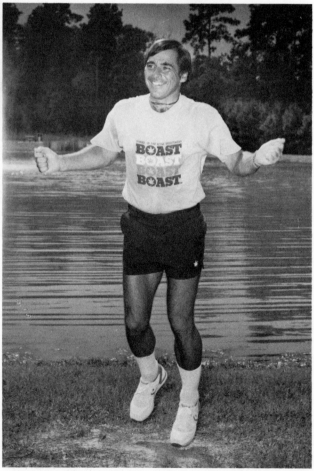

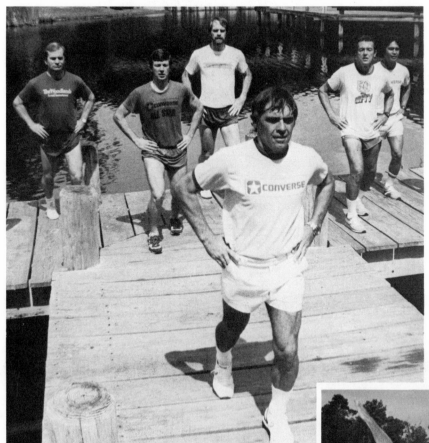

Exercise #4
Scissor Jumps #1
With hands on hips, put one foot forward and then the other, in a continuous jumping motion. You can also vary this by bouncing twice on the forward foot and then alternating. To intensify this exercise, use coordinated arm movements, such as boxer's punches.

Exercise #5
Alternate Foot Touch
While running in place, lift your legs behind you as high as possible, alternately touching the opposite heel with the opposite hand. This can also be done by bringing your feet in front of you and touching the opposite foot with the opposite hand. For a more complicated version, alternate bringing the feet in front and then in back.

Keep breathing normally!

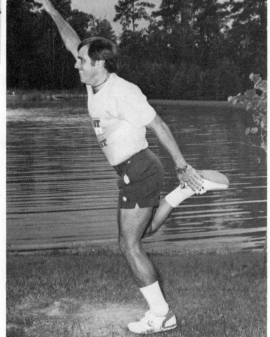

Exercise #6
Raised Thigh Jumps
Alternating legs, and
keeping your hands at
waist level, try to touch
your thigh to your hand.

To raise the intensity of
the exercise in figure 20,
try to touch your thigh to
your hand while holding
your hands higher,
thereby creating a greater
workload.

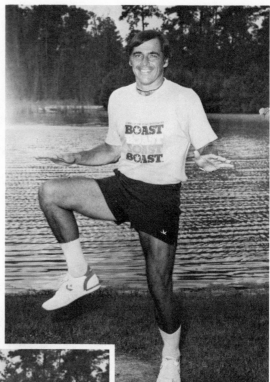

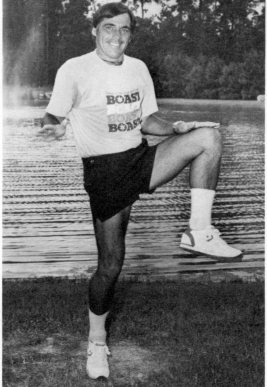

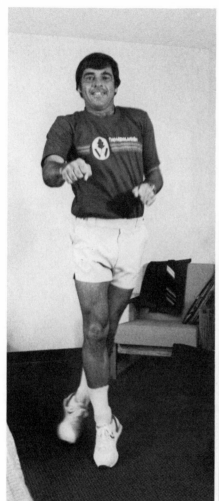

Exercise #7
Boxer's Crossover
Step #1
Hopping up and down,
alternately cross your feet
one in front of the other.
Synchronize the arms by
doing a punching motion.

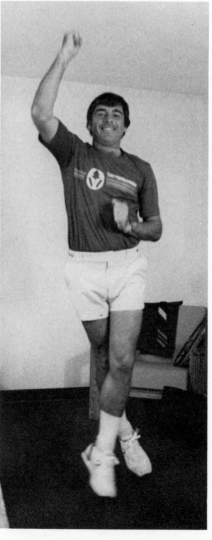

Exercise #8
Boxer's Crossover
Step #2
This is a variation of
Boxer's Crossover Step
#1. The leg motions are
the same, but the arms
are now straight up over
the head.
Note: Jog in place or
around the room while
taking your pulse. Keep
moving. Is your heart rate
too high or too low? Now
continue the workout.

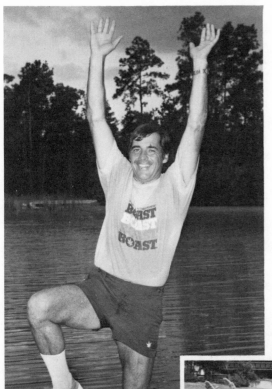

Exercise #9
Raised Arm Jump
Starting with your arms raised, hop on one foot and raise the other knee up while bringing your hands down simultaneously to meet it.

Exercise #10
Lateral Jumps
This exercise is similar to the slalom movement in skiing. Keeping your feet together, jump from side to side. It is also important that the arms move alternately up and down throughout the exercise.

Keep breathing normally!

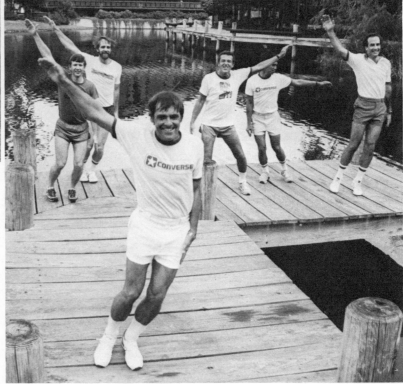

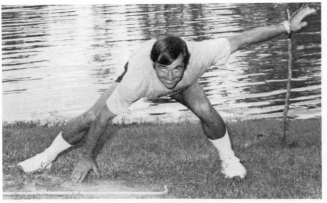

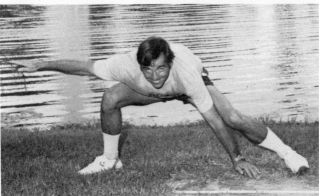

Exercise #11
Side-to-Side Lunges
Move side to side and touch the ground. It is important to stay low as you move across, and keep your head up. This is an exercise that is often used by football and basketball players and can be incorporated into an aerobics workout to give you a variation from the upright position. Because you are still moving the large muscles of the body, the heart rate can be maintained at the appropriate level for the workout.

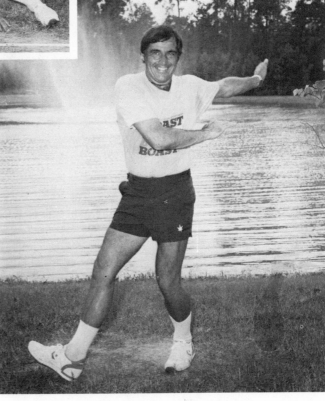

Exercise #12
Twist Jumps
Twisting from side to side, touch your heel to the ground as your foot is out. The arms swing in the opposite direction. Repeat the exercise with the opposite foot.

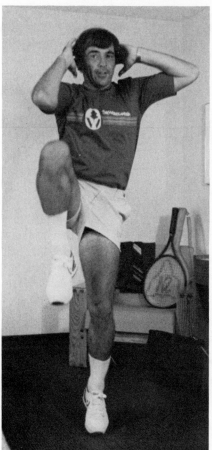

Exercise #13
Raised Knee Jumps

While keeping the upper body straight, jump on one foot and bring the knee up to the elbow. Hands are behind the head with the elbows up. It is important not to bring the head and elbow down to touch the knee. *Keep moving!*

Exercise #14
Alternate Raised Knee Jumps

Raised Knee Jumps and Alternate Raised Knee Jumps are the same, except in Alternate Raised Knee Jumps the raised knee is crossed over in front of the upper body toward the opposite elbow. Once again, keep the torso upright.

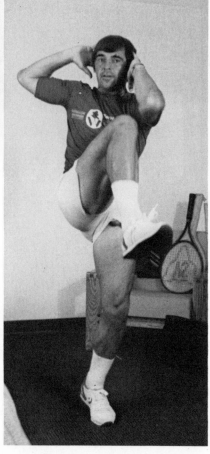

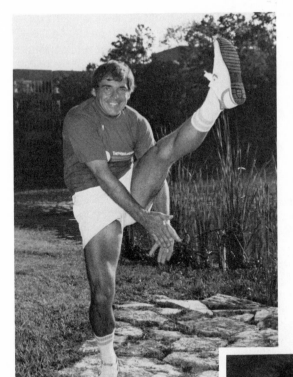

Exercise #15
High Leg Kicks—Forward
Steadily jumping on alternate legs, kick the opposite leg out in front of you, as high as possible. Try not to bend the knee. Clap your hands under your leg to maintain the height of the leg kick and the beat. If you are not very limber, kick lower. Do not strain.

Exercise #16
High Leg Kicks—Lateral
This exercise is part of a continuous movement, kicking first one leg and then the other out to the side. The objective is to kick as high as possible and keep the legs straight. Clapping your hands involves the movement of the arms and also helps with the rhythm.

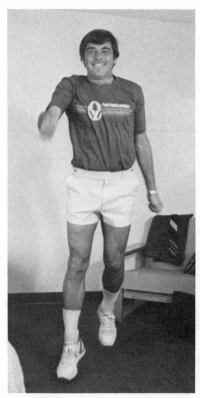

Exercise #17
Scissor Jumps #2

Put one foot forward and then the other in a continuous jumping motion. Pump the arms in an opposite pattern with the feet. There are a variety of exercises that can be incorporated into

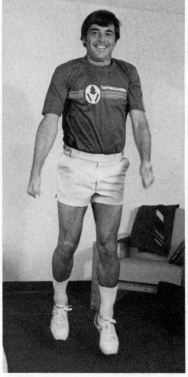

this basic movement. For example, you can do the jumping jack motion with the upper part of the body, still keeping the feet moving forward and backward.

Note: Now jog again, checking your heart rate while continuously moving. Bring your heart rate down by slowly jogging in place or around the room. You want to get the heart rate down so that cramping or pooling of blood in the legs doesn't occur while you're cooling down.

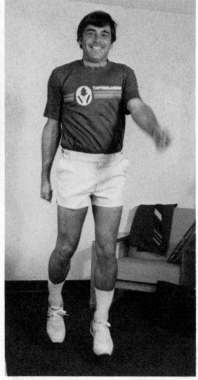

The Get-in-Shape and Maintenance Cool-down

3 MINUTES

A proper cool-down after your workout is very important. The cool-down allows your heart rate to slow down gradually and relaxes your muscles. If you don't cool down properly, your muscles may feel cramped and sore later.

Also, during the cool-down, it's a good idea to slip on your warm-up pants if you worked out in shorts.

Suggested Music

SONG TITLE	ARTIST	ALBUM TITLE
"Rainbow's End"	Sergio Mendez	*Sergio Mendez*
"Tonight I Celebrate My Love"	Roberta Flack and Peabo Bryson	*Born to Love*
"Harbor Lights"	Boz Scaggs	*Silk Degrees*
"Fire and Rain"	James Taylor	*James Taylor's Greatest Hits*
"Touch Me in the Morning"	Diana Ross	*Diana Ross's Greatest Hits*
"Three Times a Lady"	Lionel Richie	*The Best of the Commodores*
"The Wind Beneath My Wings"	Gary Morris	*Why Lady Why*

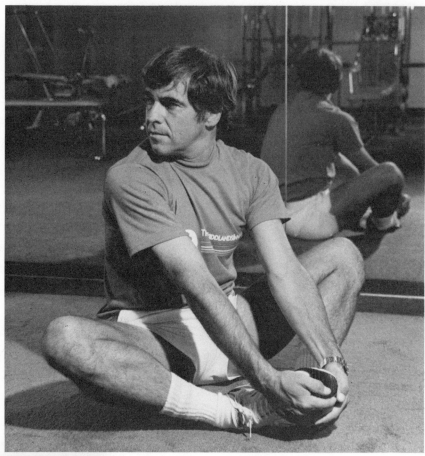

Exercise #1
Bent Knee Groin Stretch
After you have completed
the aerobics portion of
your workout, sit down,
bring the soles of your feet
together, sit up straight
with the stomach pulled
in, and look over your
right shoulder.
Note: Your breathing rate
should now be back to
normal.

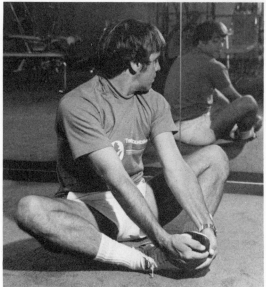

As in figure 36, repeat the
process, but this time look
over your left shoulder. A
variation of this exercise is
to bring your feet closer to
the body and try to push
the knees as close to the
floor as possible. This is
very beneficial for
stretching the inner
thighs. Keep the back
straight.

Exercise #2
Spinal Twist

In a sitting position with legs crossed, bring the left foot close to your buttocks. Cross the right leg over the left leg, keeping the knee bent. Twist the upper torso to the right as far as possible. You will benefit from this only if you feel a good stretch. Repeat the process in the opposite direction by reversing the legs and twisting in the opposite direction.

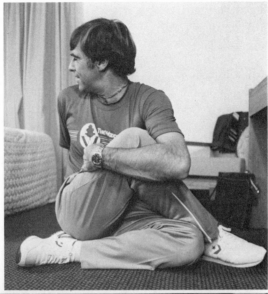

Exercise #3
Spinal Stretch

In a kneeling position, sit back on your heels. Bend forward, forehead to the ground, and extend your arms in front of you. Try to get the maximum stretch by ''walking'' your hands forward.

Exercise #4
Upper-Back Stretch

Lie down on your stomach with your feet slightly farther apart than shoulder width. Bending at the waist, walk your hands completely forward until your hips rest on the ground. Lift your head up so that you feel the stretch. The key is to have your hips on the ground. Do not do this stretch if you suffer from lower-back problems.

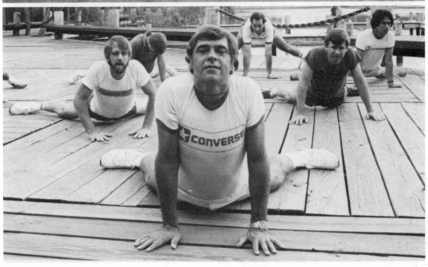

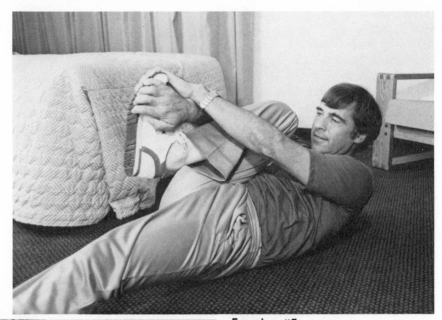

Exercise #5
Cross-Handed
Leg Stretch #1

Lie down on your back, stretching your left leg straight out. Bring your right knee to your chest, clasping the hands around the foot cross-handed. Try to bring the knee to your ear.

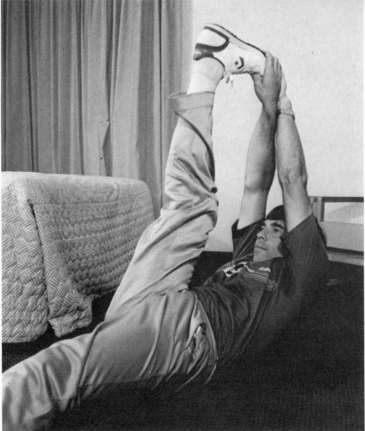

Continuing from figure 41, straighten your right leg, keeping the left leg straight. An attempt should be made to grasp the foot with the hands; if this is not possible, see figure 43.

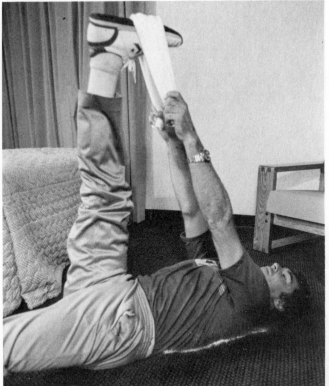

**Exercise #6
Cross-Handed
Leg Stretch #2**
Using an extension (for
example, a towel), it is
possible to keep the leg
straight. This complete
stretching of the leg is
very important during the
cool-down session.

**Exercise #7
Crossover Stretch**
While still grasping the
foot with your left hand,
cross the right leg over the
body to the floor. Every
effort should be made to
try to keep both shoulders
flat on the ground. Repeat
the process with the other
leg.

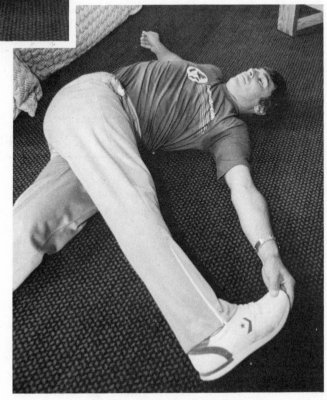

CHAPTER 11

THE ADVANCED WORKOUT

The Advanced Workout is a longer, more intense, and more thorough workout designed to get you in top physical shape and keep you there. It includes floor exercises to develop your muscular strength and endurance, which were not included in the Get-in-Shape and Maintenance Workout.

If you're in good shape already and you can do the Get-in-Shape Workout without much strain, move on to the Advanced Workout.

LENGTH OF WORKOUT: 45 minutes

FREQUENCY: 4 or 5 times a week

The Advanced Warm-Up

6 to 8 MINUTES

The warm-up exercises loosen the muscles, warm the body, and prepare the cardiovascular system for the strenuous exercise to come. They also reduce the risk of injury.

☐ If you don't have an exercise mat, lay a large towel or blanket on the floor, preferably carpeted, so you have a clean, comfortable place to exercise.

☐ Only stretch as far as you can comfortably reach. *Do not bounce* to increase your reach. Feel the stretch and then hold the position for ten to twenty seconds.

☐ Breathe normally and regularly throughout the stretches.

☐ Go through all the stretches, and if you still don't feel warm and limber, go through them once again.

Suggested Music

SONG TITLE	ARTIST	ALBUM TITLE
"Blue Bayou"	Linda Ronstadt	*Simple Dreams*
"Design for Living"	Nona Hendryx	*Nona Hendryx*
"Georgia"	Boz Scaggs	*Silk Degrees*
"Fairy Tale High"	Donna Summer	*Live and More*
"Keep It Confidential"	Nona Hendryx	*Nona Hendryx*
"Mexico"	James Taylor	*James Taylor's Greatest Hits*

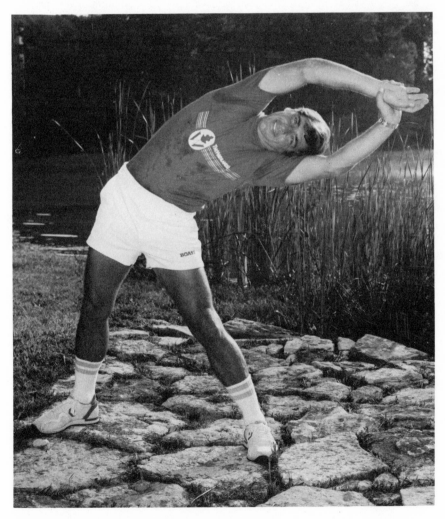

Exercise #1   Side Bends
Clasping your arms over your head, feet shoulder width apart, bend sideways at the waist as far as you can to the left, making sure you don't turn the upper torso. Keep the stomach and buttocks pulled in and bend straight to the side; then do the same exercise to the right. This is only beneficial if you stretch as far as possible. You may also rotate slowly in a circle, keeping your legs and hips in place. If you are particularly stiff, you can do Single Side Bends. Simply stretch one arm over your head while placing the other arm on your hip.

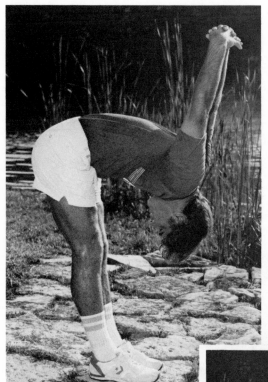

Exercise #2
Overhead Arm Stretch

With your feet about two inches apart and your legs straight, clasp your hands behind your back and bring them up as you bend forward at the waist. As your chest and arm muscles stretch out, bend a little farther forward. Do not strain.

Exercise #3
Knee Bends

With your arms straight out in front of you, squat down, keeping your back straight. Raise up on your toes and hold for a few seconds. Do not let your buttocks go any lower than the level of your knees. Deep knee bends can be dangerous.

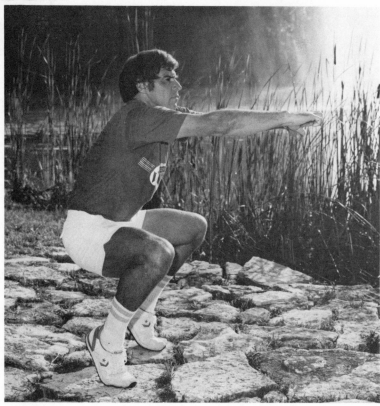

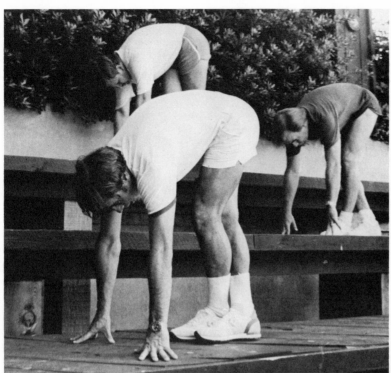

Exercise #4 Crossovers

Bending forward at the waist, try to touch your hands to the ground. Do not strain or bounce. Keeping your legs straight, cross your left foot over your right foot. Hold for a few seconds, return to a position with your feet together, and then cross your right foot over your left foot and stretch again. A lot of runners use Crossovers to stretch their hamstrings.

Exercise #5
Skier's Stretch

With your feet a little farther apart than shoulder width and your knees bent, turn your ankles out slowly and push out on your knees. This is an excellent exercise for tennis players, skiers, hockey players, or anyone involved in a sport that fosters frequent ankle injuries.

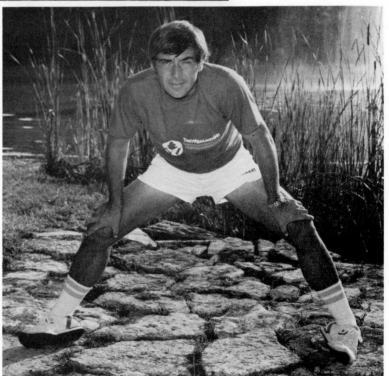

Exercise #6
Hand Walks

With your feet as wide apart as possible, walk your hands back between your legs as far as you can. Do not strain.

Keep breathing normally! Do not hold your breath.

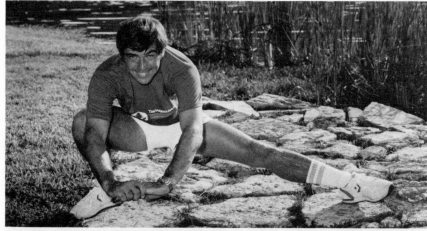

Exercise #7
Back Stretch

With your feet as wide apart as possible, cross your arms. Bending at the waist, try to touch your arms to the ground. Do not bounce! It is important to keep the legs straight.

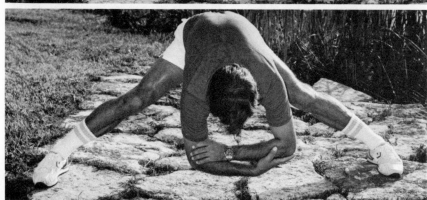

Exercise #8
Runner's Stretch

With both heels flat on the ground and your legs straight, walk your hands forward as far as you can without bringing your heels off the ground.

Exercise #9
Hurdler's Stretch

Position your left leg forward and your right leg behind. (Make sure that the top of the foot is on the ground as in the photograph.) Keep your left heel on the ground and feel the stretch in the back of your right thigh. Switch the position of your legs to stretch the left leg.

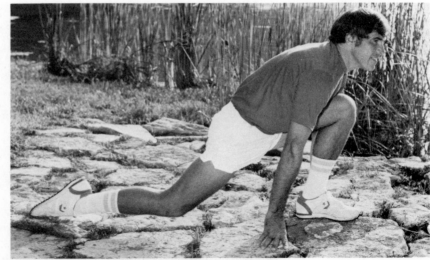

Exercise #10
Modified Hurdler's Stretch

From the position in figure 53, transfer the weight to the toes of the right leg by rocking back slowly and gently. Make sure that the left heel remains on the ground.

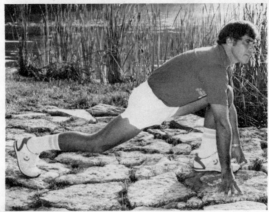

Exercise #11
Groin Stretch

With your feet as wide apart as possible, transfer your weight onto your right leg, with your toe pointing at a forty-five-degree angle. Straighten your left leg and apply gentle pressure downward on the left leg. Then switch legs and continue the exercise, transferring the weight to the left leg. This is an excellent exercise for the inside of the thigh.

THE ADVANCED
WORKOUT

85

Exercise #12
Squat Stretch
Squat down with both heels on the ground, arms out in front of you. Stretch your right leg out to one side, keeping both heels on the ground.

From figure 56, transfer the weight smoothly onto your right leg. As you transfer across, stay low. Make sure you keep both heels on the ground once the stretch is completed.

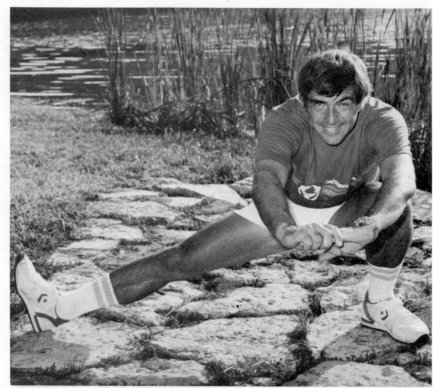

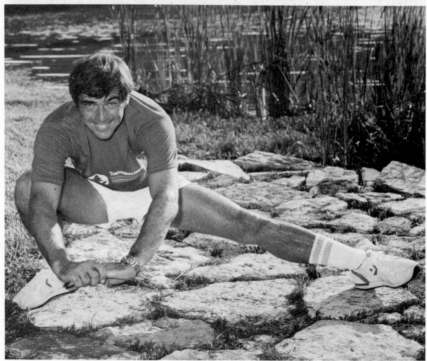

Exercise #13
Split Stretch

Sitting down, spread your legs as far apart as possible. Bend forward at the waist and grasp your toes, keeping your legs straight. If you can't reach your toes, bend as far forward as possible and flex your toes up for the same effect. If you do not feel a full stretch, then try to pull the toes toward you more. This is an excellent stretch for the calf muscles in particular.

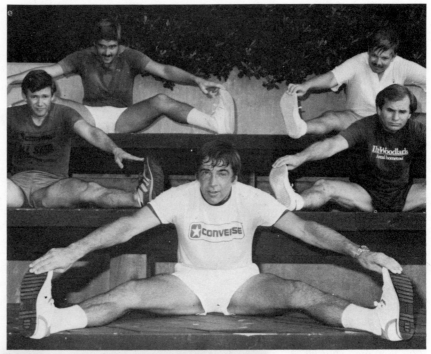

Exercise #14
Full Hamstring Stretch

In a sitting position, bring your legs together and bend forward at the waist. Keeping your knees straight, reach forward and grasp the tops of your toes. Pull the toes toward you and lift your heels off the ground. Bend your knees a little if this stretch is too difficult. Remember, keep your stomach pulled in and keep breathing.

THE ADVANCED
WORKOUT

**Exercise #15
Modified
Hamstring Stretch**
Extend your left leg in front of you. Keep your right leg bent and close to the body. Take a deep breath. While exhaling, bend forward at the waist, grasping the foot with both hands. Try to pull your chest to your thigh. If you cannot reach your foot, then grab your ankle. It is important to keep the legs straight. In the beginning, most men will have a lot of difficulty with this exercise. Gradually, greater flexibility will develop.

Now with your left leg bent back and your right leg stretched forward, bend forward at the waist, trying to grasp the bottom of your foot with both hands. Try to touch your chest to your thigh.

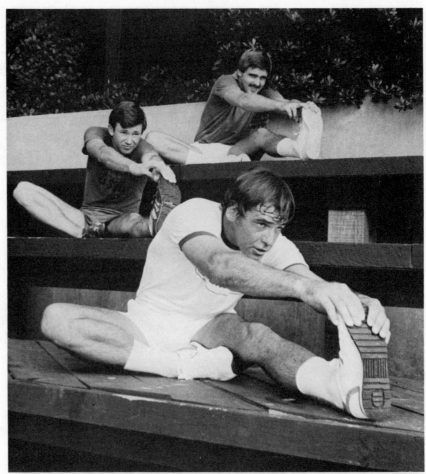

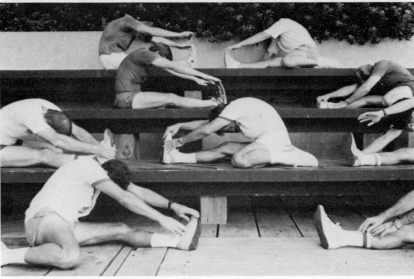

The Advanced Aerobic Exercises

20 MINUTES

The aerobic exercises are designed to build your cardiovascular fitness.

☐ In order to improve your cardiovascular fitness, you must keep moving throughout the aerobic exercises, so that your heart will continue to beat at your training rate.

☐ To make the exercises *more* strenuous, simply exaggerate all the movements of the arms and legs. Punch your fists out and then up. Kick your legs higher.

☐ Do each exercise for no more than thirty seconds. Then move on to the next exercise. As soon as you feel your muscles fatiguing, switch to another exercise.

☐ *Do not hold your breath.* It is important that you breathe deeply and regularly throughout the workout, but especially during the aerobic exercises.

☐ To ensure that you're exercising at your proper training rate throughout the aerobic exercises, take your pulse twice during this part of the workout.

Suggested Music

SONG TITLE	ARTIST	ALBUM TITLE
"The Eye of the Tiger"	Survivor	*The Eye of the Tiger*
"Walk Right Now"	The Jacksons	*Triumph*
"Gloria"	Laura Branigan	*Branigan*
"Abracadabra"	The Steve Miller Band	*Abracadabra*
"Hungry Like the Wolf"	Duran Duran	*Rio*
"Overkill"	Men at Work	*Cargo*
"One Thing Leads to Another"	The Fixx	*Reach the Beach*
"Baby Jane"	Rod Stewart	*Body Wishes*
"Physical"	Olivia Newton-John	*Physical*
"We Got the Beat"	The Go Go's	*Beauty and the Beat*
"You Should Be Dancing"	The Bee Gee's	*Bee Gee's Greatest Hits*
"We Made It"	Toto	*Toto IV*
"What a Feeling"	Irene Cara	*Flashdance*

"Space Age Love"	A Flock of Seagulls	*A Flock of Seagulls*
"Bad Girls"	Donna Summer	*Bad Girls*
"She Works Hard for the Money"	Donna Summer	*She Works Hard for the Money*
"Beat It"	Michael Jackson	*Thriller*
"Billie Jean"	Michael Jackson	*Thriller*
"P.Y.T."	Michael Jackson	*Thriller*

Exercise #1
Resting Kick
With your hands on your hips, lean slightly back and jump steadily on one leg and kick with the other. Alternate legs every two jumps.
Note: If you get too tired to continue the workout, use the Resting Kick or simply jog in place to catch your breath; then continue the workout. To vary this exercise you can also use arm movements, such as boxer's punches, while you do the kick.

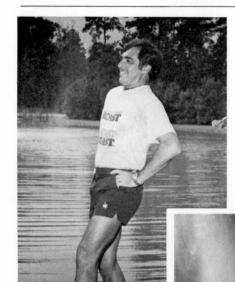

Exercise #2
Jump and Twist
Twist from side to side on both feet while swinging the arms on the opposite side of the body.

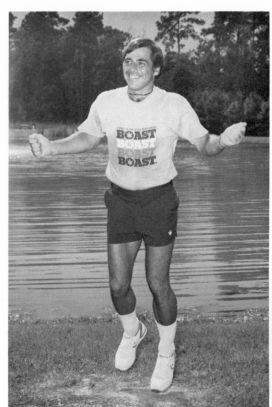

Exercise #3
Skipping Rope
This exercise is just like skipping rope, but without the rope. There are innumerable variations of this aerobic movement (for example, hopping twice on one foot and alternating to the other foot, keeping the movement continuous).

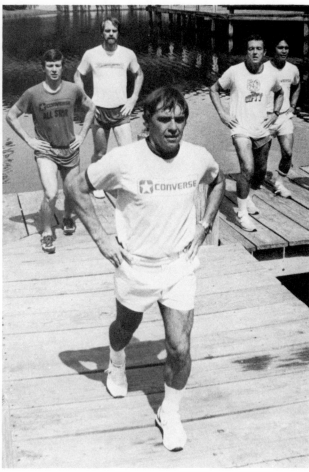

Exercise #4
Scissor Jumps #1
With hands on hips, put one foot forward and then the other, in a continuous jumping motion. You can also vary this by bouncing twice on the forward foot and then alternating. To intensify this exercise, use coordinated arm movements, such as boxer's punches.

Exercise #5
Alternate Foot Touch
While running in place, lift your legs behind you as high as possible, alternately touching the opposite heel with the opposite hand. This can also be done by bringing your feet in front of you and touching the opposite foot with the opposite hand. For a more complicated version, alternate bringing the feet in front and then in back.

Keep breathing normally!

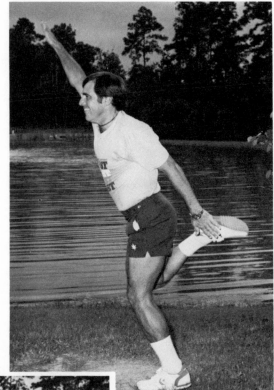

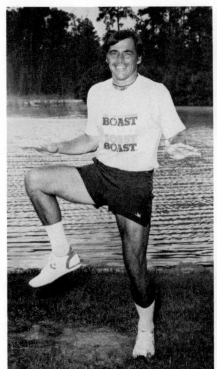

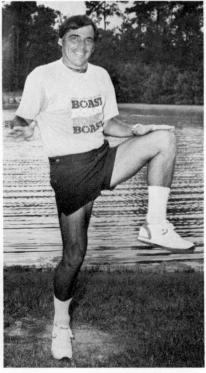

Exercise #6
Raised Thigh Jumps
Alternating legs, and keeping your hands at waist level, try to touch your thigh to your hand.

To raise the intensity of the exercise in figure 67, try to touch your thigh to your hand while holding your hands higher, thereby creating a greater workload.

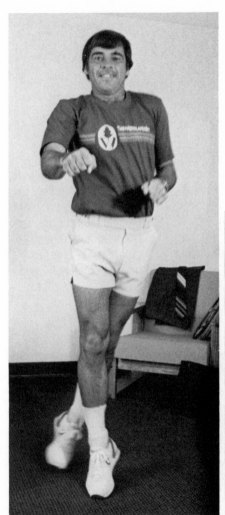

Exercise #7
Boxer's
Crossover Step #1
Hopping up and down, alternately cross your feet one in front of the other. Synchronize the arms by doing a punching motion.

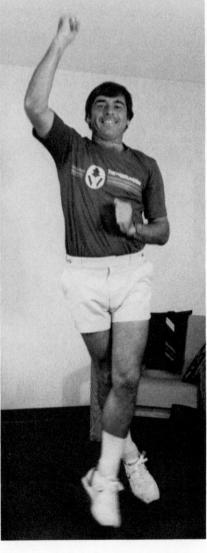

Exercise #8
Boxer's
Crossover Step #2
This is a variation of Boxer's Crossover Step #1. The leg motions are the same, but the arms are now straight up over the head.
Note: Jog in place or around the room while taking your pulse. Keep moving. Is your heart rate too high or too low? Now continue the workout.

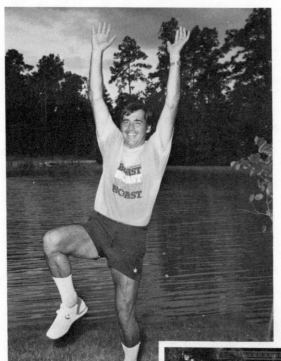

Exercise #9
Raised Arm Jump
Starting with your arms raised, hop on one foot and raise the other knee up while bringing your hands down simultaneously to meet it.

Exercise #10
Lateral Jumps
This exercise is similar to the slalom movement in skiing. Keeping your feet together, jump from side to side. It is also important that the arms move alternately up and down throughout the exercise.
Keep breathing normally!

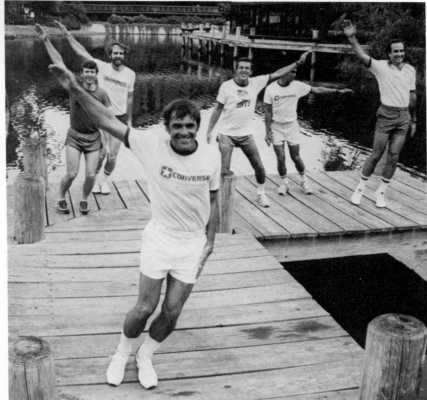

Exercise #11
Side-to-Side Lunges

Move side to side and touch the ground. It is important to stay low as you move across, and keep your head up. This is an exercise that is often used by football and basketball players and can be incorporated into an aerobics workout to give you a variation from the upright position. Because you are still moving the large muscles of the body, the heart rate can be maintained at the appropriate level for the workout.

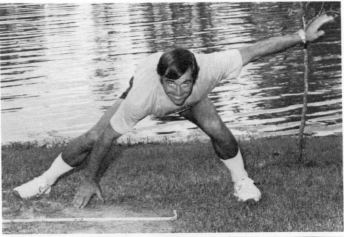

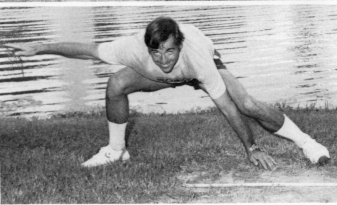

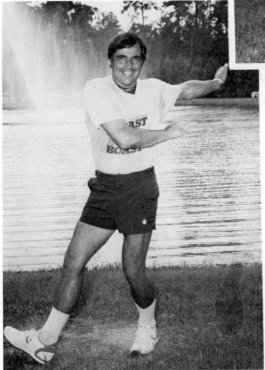

Exercise #12
Twist Jumps

Twisting from side to side, touch your heel to the ground as your foot is out. The arms swing in the opposite direction. Repeat the exercise with the opposite foot.

THE ADVANCED
WORKOUT

95

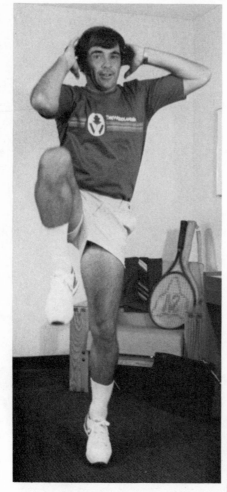

Exercise #13
Raised Knee Jumps
While keeping the upper
body straight, jump on
one foot and bring the
knee up to the elbow.
Hands are behind the head
with the elbows up. It is
important not to bring the
head and elbow down to
touch the knee. *Keep
moving!*

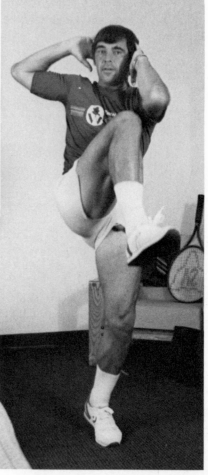

Exercise #14
Alternate Raised
Knee Jumps
Raised Knee Jumps and
Alternate Raised Knee
Jumps are the same
except in Alternate Raised
Knee Jumps the raised
knee is crossed over in
front of the upper body
toward the opposite
elbow. Once again, keep
the torso upright.

Exercise #16
High Leg Kicks—Lateral

This exercise is part of a continuous movement, kicking first one leg and then the other out to the side. The objective is to kick as high as possible and keep the legs straight. Clapping your hands involves the movement of the arms and also helps with the rhythm.

Exercise #15
High Leg Kicks—Forward

Steadily jumping on alternate legs, kick the opposite leg out in front of you as high as possible. Try not to bend the knee. Clap your hands under your leg to maintain the height of the leg kick and the beat. If you are not very limber, kick lower. Do not strain.

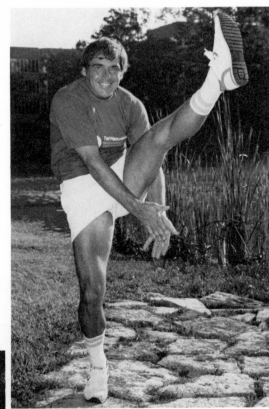

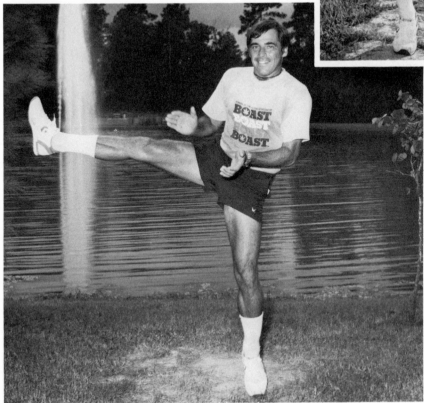

Exercise #17
Scissor Jumps #2
Put one foot forward and then the other in a continuous jumping motion. Pump the arms in an opposite pattern with the feet. There are a variety of exercises that can be incorporated into this basic movement. For example, you can do the jumping jack motion with the upper part of the body, still keeping the feet moving forward and backward.

Note: Now jog again, checking your heart rate while continuously moving. Bring your heart rate down by slowly jogging in place or around the room. You want to get the heart rate down so that cramping or pooling of blood in the legs doesn't occur while you're doing the floor exercises. Now on to the floor work.

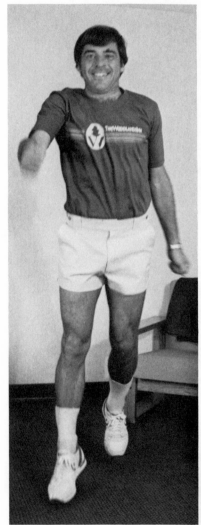
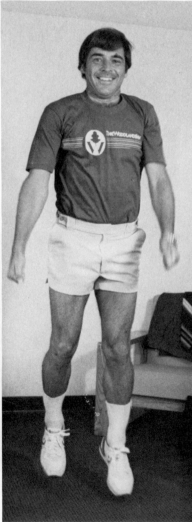
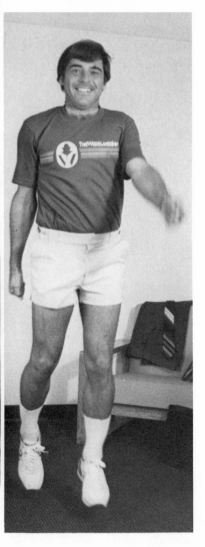

The Advanced Floor Exercises

15 MINUTES

The floor exercises are designed to burn away your intramuscular fat and build muscular strength and muscular endurance.

☐ Do as many repetitions of each exercise as you can. The number of repetitions to be performed is suggested, but they are meant to be a guide only. Do only as many repetitions as you can without hurting.

☐ Do each exercise as smoothly as you can. Do not jerk the muscles.

☐ Squeeze your buttocks whenever possible during the floor exercises. This helps the other muscle groups to work harder.

Suggested Music

SONG TITLE	ARTIST	ALBUM TITLE
"Fame"	Irene Cara	*Fame*
"Africa"	Toto	*Toto IV*
"Gloria"	Laura Branigan	*Branigan*
"Physical"	Olivia Newton-John	*Physical*
"She Works Hard for the Money"	Donna Summer	*She Works Hard for the Money*
"Dreams"	Fleetwood Mac	*Rumours*

AEROBIC WORKOUT
BOOK FOR MEN

Exercise #1
Scissor Kicks
Repetitions: 30 (two
Scissor Kicks equals
one repetition)
Muscles worked:
abdominals, inner thigh
    Sit down and lean back
with your hands on the
floor behind you. Stretch
the legs straight out in
front of you. In a
continuous movement,
spread the legs wide apart
and then bring them
together, crossing one
foot over the other. Point
the toes for 10 counts,
then flex the foot for 10
counts, then point the toes
for the last 10 counts.
Remember to keep the
stomach muscles held in
and don't hold your
breath.

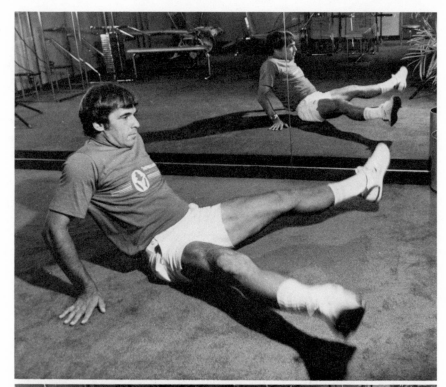

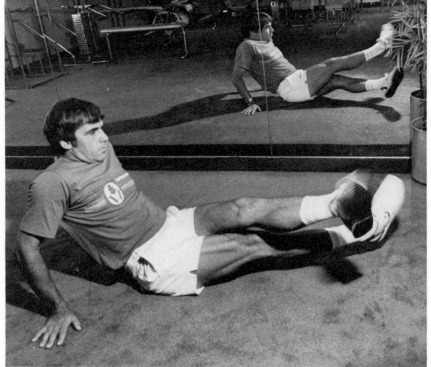

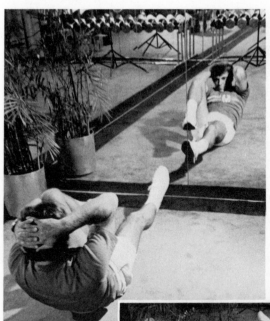

Exercise #2
Elbow-to-Knee Situps

Repetitions: 32

Muscles worked: upper and lower abdominals

Lie on your back with your hands clasped behind your head. Bring your left elbow to your right knee, then back down and bring your right elbow to your left knee. Make sure your upper body is coming off the ground so that the stomach is getting a workout. Nothing is gained by only moving the elbows. As this exercise gets faster, the tendency is to bend the neck and head forward so that there is a lesser distance between the elbow and knee. That's cheating! Make the stomach work.

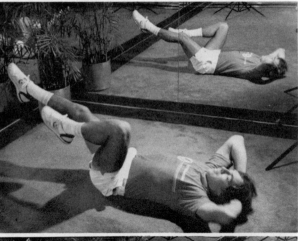

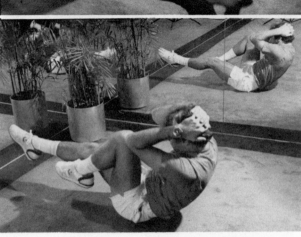

Exercise #3
Alternating
Elbow-to-Knee Situps

Repetitions: 32

Muscles worked: upper and lower abdominals, obliques

Lie on your back with your hands behind your head. Stretch one leg out straight and raise it 16 to 18 inches off the ground. The other leg is bent, with the knee in toward the stomach. Alternating elbows, try to touch one, then the other elbow to the raised knee. Do not let the straight leg touch the ground or get raised too high. Also, make sure the lower back stays flat on the floor, and the stomach muscles are held in tightly. When done correctly, your stomach muscles will be worked strenuously.

AEROBIC WORKOUT
BOOK FOR MEN

Exercise #4
Back Leg Lifts
Repetitions: 20 on each
side
Muscles worked:
hamstrings

On your hands and
knees, stretch one leg
straight out behind you.
Raise and lower it,
keeping the muscles taut
and the leg straight. Do
10 repetitions with the
toes pointed and 10
repetitions with the foot
flexed. Switch legs. Don't
jerk the leg up and down;
keep the movement
controlled.

If you need to
strengthen your upper
body, do some pushups
now. Continue until your
arms get tired.

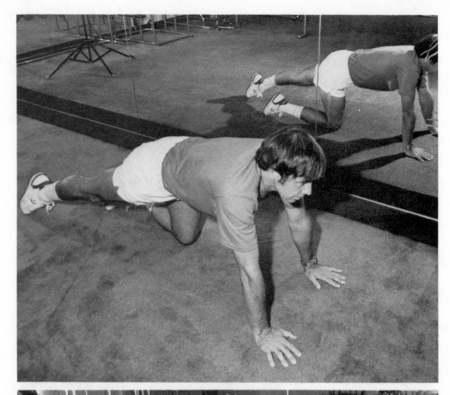

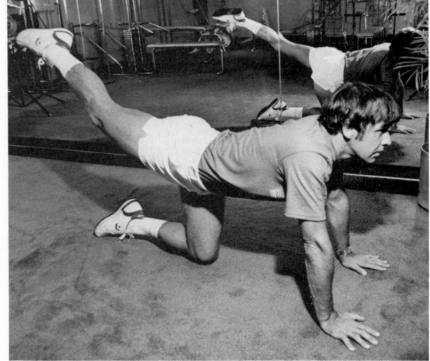

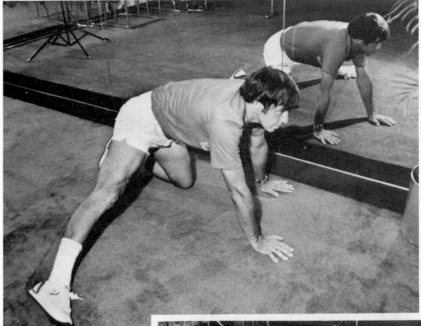

Exercise #5
Side Leg Lifts
Repetitions: 20 on each
side
Muscles worked: gluteus
maximus, inner thigh

Get down on your
hands and knees and
stretch one leg out to the
side. Flex the foot and
keep the leg straight.
Raise the leg up and
down, but never let the
foot touch the ground.
Make sure the leg stays
out to the side. Keep the
hips parallel to the floor.
Just lift the leg. As you
gain strength, you'll be
able to raise your leg just
about level with your hip.

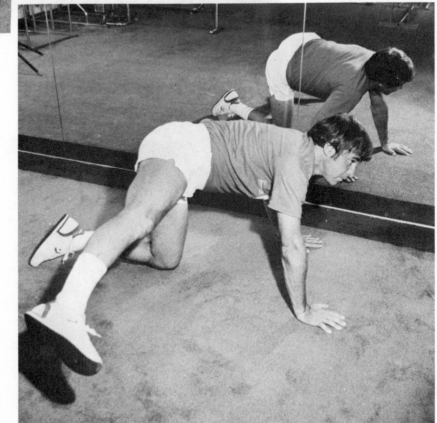

Exercise #6
Flutter Kicks

Repetitions: 20 on each side

Muscles worked: inner thigh, hips

Lie on your side, with your head propped up on your hand. Kick your feet in a fluttering motion, making sure they are not touching the ground. Keep it up at a fast pace. Roll over to change sides.

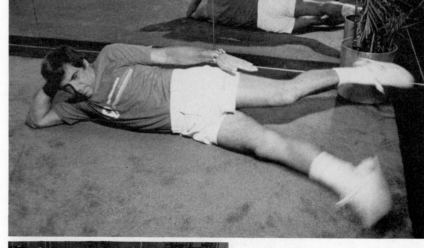

Exercise #7   Leg Lifts

Repetitions: 30 on each side

Muscles worked: inner thigh, hips, buttocks

Lie on your side, propped up on your elbow if you like. Keeping your body and legs straight, raise and lower the top leg while flexing the foot. Height is not the object. Keep all the muscles in the buttocks and legs tight. Switch legs by rolling over on your other side.

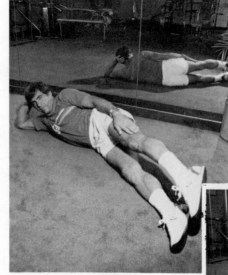

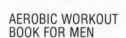

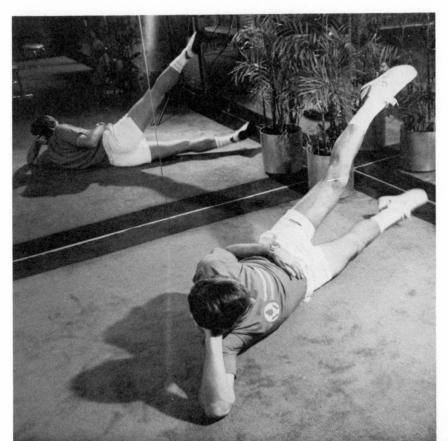

Exercise #8
Scissor Lifts
Repetitions: 15 on each side
Muscles worked: inner and outer thighs

Lie on your side and rest your head on your hand. Keeping your top leg raised as straight as possible, lift your lower leg up to touch the upper leg. This is a continuous up-and-down motion of the lower leg *only*. Try to remember not to bend at the waist or bend the knees. After at least 15 leg lifts, roll over and repeat the exercise, raising and lowering the opposite leg.

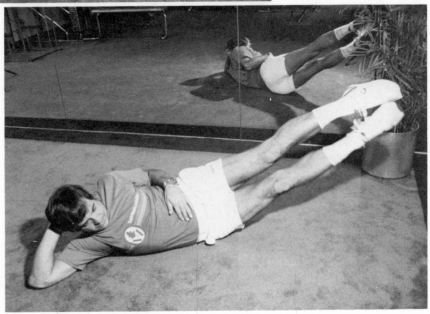

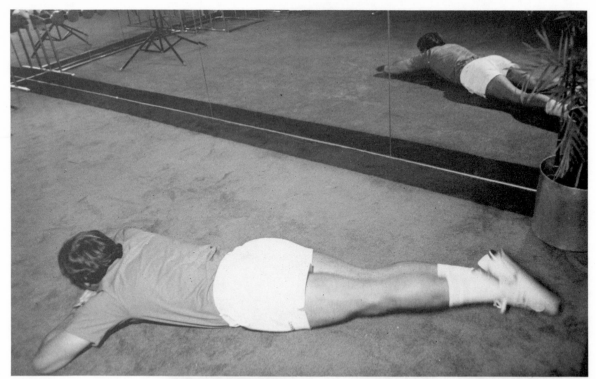

Exercise #9
Leg Extensions

Repetitions: 10 on each leg

Muscles worked: buttocks, back of thigh

Lie flat on your stomach and rest your chin on your hands. Keeping your hips on the ground, raise and lower one leg. Make sure the legs stay straight and the muscles in the buttocks and leg are taut. Once again, height is not that important. Alternate legs after 10 repetitions. Again, do not get carried away with the music and jerk your leg back too violently. You could injure your lower back.

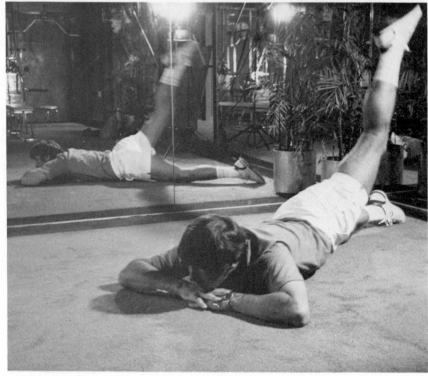

The Advanced Cool-down

4 to 6 MINUTES

A proper cool-down after your workout is extremely important. The cool-down allows your heart rate to slow down gradually and relaxes your muscles. If you don't cool down properly, your muscles may feel cramped and sore later.

Also, during the cool-down, it's a good idea to slip on your warm-up pants if you worked out in shorts.

Suggested Music

SONG TITLE	ARTIST	ALBUM TITLE
"Rainbow's End"	Sergio Mendez	*Sergio Mendez*
"Tonight I Celebrate My Love"	Roberta Flack and Peabo Bryson	*Born to Love*
"Harbor Lights"	Boz Scaggs	*Silk Degrees*
"Fire and Rain"	James Taylor	*James Taylor's Greatest Hits*
"Touch Me in the Morning"	Diana Ross	*Diana Ross's Greatest Hits*
"Three Times a Lady"	Lionel Richie	*The Best of the Commodores*
"The Wind Beneath My Wings"	Gary Morris	*Why Lady Why*

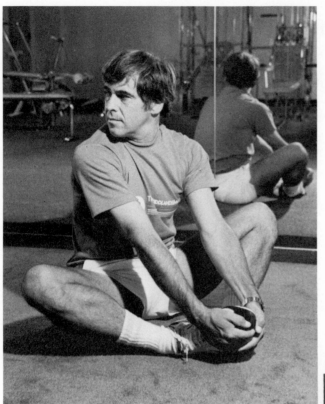

Exercise #1
Bent Knee Groin Stretch

After you have completed the aerobics portion of your workout, sit down, bring the soles of your feet together, sit up straight with the stomach pulled in, and look over your right shoulder.

As in figure 99, repeat the process, but this time look over your left shoulder. A variation of this exercise is to bring your feet closer to the body and try to push the knees as close to the floor as possible. This is very beneficial for stretching the inner thighs. Keep the back straight.

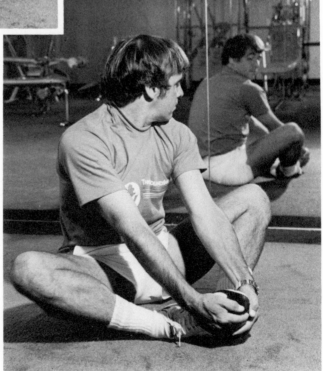

Exercise #2
Spinal Twist

In a sitting position with legs crossed, bring the left foot close to your buttocks. Cross the right leg over the left leg, keeping the knee bent. Twist the upper torso to the right as far as possible. You will benefit from this only if you feel a good stretch. Repeat the process in the opposite direction by reversing the legs and twisting in the opposite direction.

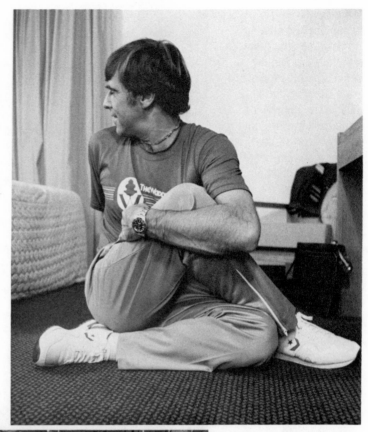

Exercise #3
Spinal Stretch

In a kneeling position, sit back on your heels. Bend forward, forehead to the ground, and extend your arms in front of you. Try to get the maximum stretch by ''walking'' your hands forward.

Exercise #4
Upper-Back Stretch

Lie down on your stomach with your feet slightly farther apart than shoulder width. Bending at the waist, walk your hands completely forward until your hips rest on the ground. Lift your head up so that you feel the stretch. The key is to have your hips on the ground. Do not do this stretch if you suffer from lower-back problems.

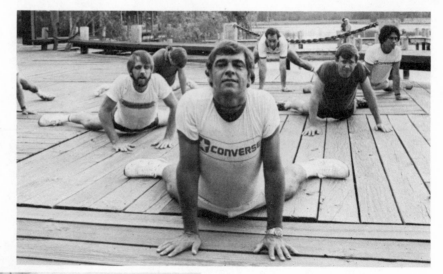

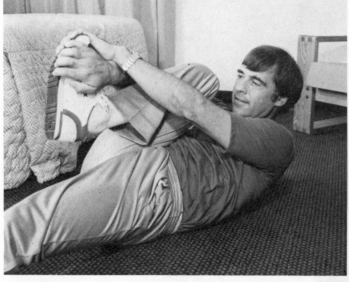

Exercise #5
Cross-Handed
Leg Stretch #1

Lie down on your back, stretching your left leg straight out. Bring your right knee to your chest, clasping the hands around the foot cross-handed. Try to bring the knee to your ear.

Continuing from figure 104, straighten your right leg, keeping the left leg straight. An attempt should be made to grasp the foot with the hands; if this is not possible, see figure 106.

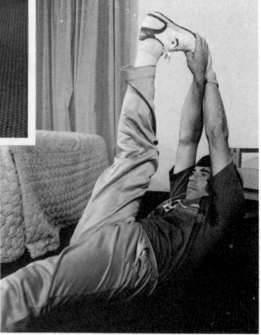

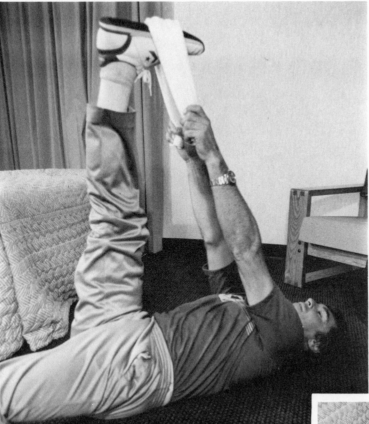

Exercise #6
Cross-Handed
Leg Stretch #2

Using an extension (for example, a towel) it is possible to keep the leg straight. This complete stretching of the leg is very important during the cool-down session.

Exercise #7
Crossover Stretch

While still grasping the foot with your left hand, cross the right leg over the body to the floor. Every effort should be made to try to keep both shoulders flat on the ground. Repeat the process with the other leg.

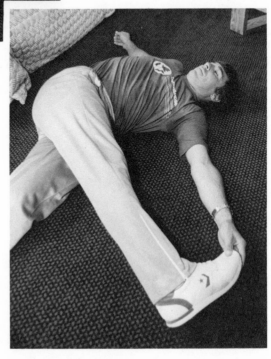

Exercise #8   The Plough

(A yoga stretch)
Lie on your back, bring
your knees into your
chest, then slowly raise
them over your head.
Attempt to touch the toes
to the ground. It may be
helpful to support the
lower back with your
hands if you have never
done this exercise before.
To release, slowly lower
your legs overhead,
keeping the thighs close to
the chest. Then slide the
legs to the floor. Now
relax your whole body.

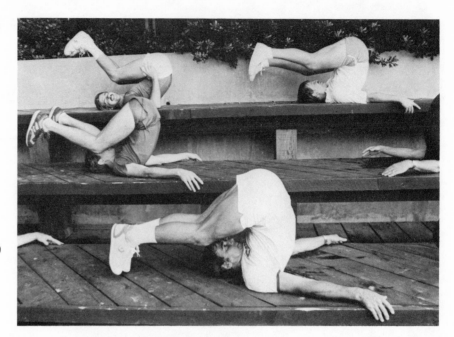

CHAPTER 12

THE SUPER WORKOUT
FOR THE SUPER ATHLETE

An athlete trained by aerobics gains a blend of speed, coordination, and endurance that can give him an edge in almost any sport. The Super Workout is a sports-conditioning program designed to get the serious athlete into training-camp fitness for competition. It is geared for an athlete involved in high school, university, or professional competition. It is not a casual program. Only undertake the Super Workout if you are already in superb condition and have some specific, sports-related goal in mind.

The Super Workout

Basically, the Super Workout is the same as the Advanced Workout except that you should exercise with a training heart rate of 85 percent of your maximum heart rate. If you become winded or fatigued, you are not ready for this workout. Continue to exercise at the training heart rate for the Advanced Workout until you can do it with relative ease. The increase of 5 percent in your training rate is an enormous one at that pace—so be careful. If you encounter any symptoms of heart strain, such as pain or tightness in the chest or dizziness, stop exercising immediately.

Weights

Ordinarily, the weight of your own body as you do your workout is sufficient to build muscular strength and endurance. But if you are

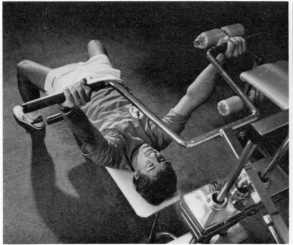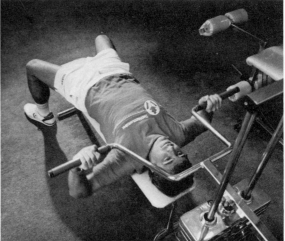

There is a lot of equipment on the market today that can do nearly everything when it comes time to selective muscle exercising. These machines are excellent for muscle building and toning, but they cannot benefit you aerobically. They won't help take off your fat.

very fit or you want to gain added strength for some specific, sports-related reason, the exercises may not be strenuous enough for you. Adding weights to your workout can help.

One way you can increase your training heart rate and further develop your strength is by doing the workout while using hand and foot weights weighing anywhere from one to ten pounds. Several companies now make weights that attach conveniently to your wrists and ankles. They are available at most sporting goods stores.

Doing the aerobic exercises and the floor exercises with these weights can increase your strength tremendously. But if you want to build even greater upper-body strength, I suggest you find a good weight-training program, such as the Nautilus program, with instructors schooled in strength training.

Let me emphasize, however, that the Super Workout is not a body-building program. It is a workout designed to get you in superior physical condition. Body building and weight lifting do not, by themselves, get you fit or healthy. They build up your muscle tissue and those muscles may be loaded with fat. Body building does little for your heart and lungs.

Jumping Rope and Wind Sprints

The Super Workout and a well-planned weight-training program are all you need to develop all five elements of physical fitness to their greatest potential. But two other exercises also can be beneficial: jumping rope and wind sprints.

Jumping rope is ideal for developing hand, foot, and eye coordination. Coordination is important to an athlete because it enables him to perform with an economy of motion. Every movement of his body is directed toward his objective, whether it's hitting a ball or jumping a hurdle. If your hips are going one way and your shoulders another, you will lose power and speed. Better coordination also helps prevent injuries.

I suggest that you do three sets of one hundred jumps, every other day.

Wind sprints can help build your oxygen uptake and lung capacity and increase the glucose-burning efficiency in your muscles. I recommend that you do a series of five wind sprints of forty yards apiece, performed with thirty seconds of rest between each sprint. Warm up by stretching and jogging briefly before doing sprints.

Eating Before a Competition

For fifteen years, my meal before every tennis match has been spaghetti or some other form of pasta, because it is a source of complex carbohydrates. This breaks down slowly into energy-producing glycogen.

For me, the best time to eat this plate of pasta is about two hours before a match. Then I know that when the match starts I will have energy, but won't feel sluggish and full. Because metabolism rates vary, do some personal experimenting to determine your best pregame mealtime.

PART FIVE

MAKING YOUR WORKOUT WORK FOR YOU

CHAPTER 13

STICKING WITH YOUR WORKOUT

Make a Commitment to Your Fitness

There are a million excuses to skip your workout—it's your birthday, you overdid it at the party last night, you've got too much work to do, your kid's graduating, the car won't start—the list is endless! But if you're going to succeed at fitness, you've got to make a commitment to your workout. To most of us that probably sounds like a jail sentence. But don't let it scare you off. It's not as hard as it seems to stick with a regular exercise program.

But first you've got to ignore all those bad things you've heard about exercise like "no pain, no gain." In truth, most of this nonsense has come from those who exercise the most. They make it sound as if you've got to dread exercise before it will do you any good.

If you give me twenty minutes of your life every other day for a month, I promise you'll have a whole new outlook on exercise. By giving you some simple ideas and techniques that will help you stick to your program, I believe I can turn your attitude around so that you will begin to love exercise—and the healthy body that exercise creates.

Age and Fitness

One of the major obstacles to achieving fitness is the attitude in our society that the older you get, the more out of shape you get. They tell you your legs are going to go. Your eyes are going to go. It's as if there's some rule that when you lose your hair, you're supposed to acquire a big gut.

Unfortunately, most middle-aged people (and some in their thirties) seem to be swayed by this "I'm too old to exercise" propaganda. Age becomes an excuse for inactivity. They don't dare test themselves because they might strain something. This is nonsense. In truth, the older you get, the more you need exercise.

Exercise is a lifetime commitment. In fact, you must become more committed as you get older. You must have a greater responsibility to your body and your health. As you grow older you can't get away with the same bad habits you had when you were young and expect to maintain your health.

Professor Per-Olof Astrand of Sweden, an authority on health, has stated. "If two 50-year olds are identical in endowment but one is trained (i.e., systematically exercised) and the other untrained, then the trained person would have an oxygen uptake ability—and maximum motor power—on the same level as the untrained person had around the age of 35 to 40. In other words, moderate training can lead to a ten-to-fifteen-year biological rejuvenation."[13]

Get Through the First Two Weeks

Studies have shown that most people who start an exercise program quit within the first five days. There's a very good reason for this attrition rate.

After the first couple of exercise sessions, the body feels an elation from the sheer thrill of having the blood circulating again. Most people report feeling this "high" during the first week. But after that, for the next week or so, there's a letdown and the exercise can seem like pure drudgery. You're not losing any weight, your muscles are sore and tired, and the workout seems like a big chore.

After that initial two weeks, however, people once again start to feel elated after exercise. The exercise becomes easier, even though you're working harder. Also, dramatic weight losses are reported. After that, it's easy to stay with your workout.

When I first started working out, I made a firm commitment for two weeks. At five-thirty every afternoon I had a class, and no matter how important the phone call or the person, I never let anything interrupt my workout. Not only did this commitment help me stick with my workout, but it also spilled over to other parts of my life. I began to see that if I concentrated on one thing, really gave my all, really committed my time and myself to one thing at one time, I got much more done and I did it better.

It was only because I made my workout a priority that I was able to show up every day. And I'll never regret that decision.

Whether you get together with someone or exercise alone, pick a time and a day and commit yourself for two weeks. You'll be hooked on exercise at the end of that time, and then it'll be pure enjoyment— not something you think about with dread, but something you look forward to. It will simply become a part of your daily routine.

Become Exercise Conscious

For most of us, getting in shape means a regular exercise routine and a good diet. But there's a third important ingredient that most of us forget about—state of mind. If you're going to make a permanent change from the habits that got you fat and flabby to the habits of a healthy life, you've got to change your whole way of thinking. You've got to become "exercise conscious."

My life changed completely when I became exercise conscious. When I was young, I loved sports, not exercise. Every exercise I did was geared to enable me to perform better in the hockey rink, on the football field, or on the tennis court. But I wasn't at all concerned about my health.

Even my education as a physiology major did not really get through to me. I knew how the human body was supposed to work and the part that exercise played in health. But I did not understand the true importance of fitness. If I had, I would have exercised properly.

Exercise can't be just something you do on weekends or once a month. It must become as integral to your life as eating and sleeping and working. And, believe me, if you begin to exercise, and stick with it for long enough, you will understand how important and necessary regular exercise is to the quality of your life. The added energy you will have translates into that greater zest for life that we all search for. Before long you'll begin to wonder how you ever lived without regular exercise. When you reach that understanding, you will be exercise conscious. You'll see that exercise is more than shaping up to look good or to lose weight. It's as important as eating and sleeping.

The first step in becoming exercise conscious is to start thinking like a fit person. Psychological testing has shown that a person's image improves with a regular exercise program. A man who is physically fit usually has a better outlook and more self-confidence. You'll learn to relax and that will enable you to cope with the stress of daily living. Also, you will sleep better and work better—get more done with less fatigue. In other words, the more you exercise, the better you'll feel and the more you'll want to exercise.

The second step in becoming exercise conscious is to start integrating exercise into your daily life. Your whole life should be geared to physical activity—rather than avoidance of activity. Fitness is determined by what you do throughout the day—working, eating, and playing—not just how you exercise during a workout.

Make up your mind that you're going to start doing things for yourself. First of all, eliminate most of the mechanized aspects of your modern life. When you have a chance to do something manually, do it —whether it's walking up the stairs or to the corner for the paper instead of driving. Avoid the easy way. Take every opportunity that comes your way during the day to exercise your heart, lungs, and muscles—even when you're not in the gym or on the court.

There are hundreds of opportunities to exercise throughout the day. Although they may seem insignificant taken by themselves, over the course of a month or a year or a lifetime, they can make the difference between a healthy, active life and one plagued by illness.

From the moment you wake up in the morning, think exercise. Take a big long stretch, pull your knees to your chest, reach with your toes to the ceiling. When you're up, get your blood pumping right away with some easy waist and knee bends and arm rotations. Towel yourself off vigorously after a shower, stand while you dress, stretch to tie your shoes.

When you're at work, stretch out several times at your desk during the course of the work day. Get up and walk to the water cooler. Take all calls standing up, and if you want to talk to a colleague in another office down the hall, don't call him, walk over to his office and talk. Use the stairs rather than the elevator whenever possible.

For lunch go to a restaurant you have to walk a good distance to. If your office is too far from home to walk or jog to work, use a parking lot a half dozen blocks away and walk the rest of the way.

These steps may seem trivial and silly until you realize that a secretary who switches from a manual to an electric typewriter will gain six pounds a year, if she changes nothing else in her life.

When you get home from that tense day at the office, play with your kids. If they need someone to throw the ball around with, grab a glove. Help your wife with dinner; volunteer to peel the potatoes. Preparing dinner can actually be relaxing; it can take your mind off work and get your stomach ready for a pleasant meal. After dinner, walk the dog or take a stroll with your wife or girl friend.

In fact, if you've been out of shape for a long time, taking regular brisk walks is a great way to get started exercising and could be all you need to raise your heart to its training level. For a while, those evening walks with your wife or girl friend could serve as your aerobic workout.

Walking is excellent exercise if you keep up a brisk pace. And just about everyone can do it, from a cardiac patient right out of the hospital to an eighty-year-old grandmother.

Take every opportunity to walk rather than ride—to the store, to the mailbox, to the tennis courts. Every time you start up the car for a short errand, you're not only wasting gas, but your fitness as well.

Find the Right Time to Exercise

Check your daily schedule to determine the most convenient time for your workout. You must be willing to designate a specific time for exercise at least every other day. Finding the time in a busy day is not as hard as it looks at first if you really know yourself and your habits. When do you feel like exercising the most? Perhaps, a little experimenting will help you decide. It doesn't matter what time you pick, as long as it helps you stick with your workout.

Some people like to exercise first thing in the morning. They get their exercise out of the way so they feel good about themselves and free to tackle the rest of the day knowing they've taken care of their bodies.

Other people, however, can't get going for hours; the thought of a vigorous workout early in the morning fills them with dread. If you're one of these people, don't let those morning folks make you feel guilty. Exercise when it's right for you.

Lunch hour is also a popular time for working out. Not only is it convenient for people who have a place to work out near their offices, but it fits nicely into a preset discipline. Thanks to your boss, your lunch hour comes every day at a specific time—whether you like it or not. If you get into the habit of exercising at lunchtime, your self-discipline is helped along by this regimen.

Another advantage of a lunchtime workout is that vigorous exercise tends to suppress the appetite. After a heavy workout, you're just not going to feel like eating as much as you normally would. And that's great for your waist.

One warning though: never eat immediately before you exercise. Wait at least one hour after a heavy meal before exercising strenuously. The heart pumps blood to the stomach to help digestion after you eat. If you exercise on a full stomach, the blood will be diverted to muscles in the rest of your body, resulting in stomach cramps due to a lack of oxygen.

Many people like to exercise after work because it helps them get rid of all the nervous tension that builds up during the day. Instead of coming home and drinking a couple of martinis, they exercise.

Some people choose to exercise before bedtime because it makes them feel relaxed and drowsy, and it helps their insomnia. Most of you will find, however, that the late evening is not a good time for your workout because exercise often has a stimulating effect. But if it works for you, by all means, exercise before you go to bed.

One warning about exercising at night: for some reason it seems to encourage quitting. The dropout rate among those who exercise in the morning is less than 30 percent. Among those who exercise in the afternoon or evening, it's more than 60 percent. Perhaps it's easier to find excuses not to exercise at night: you had a late dinner and you're too full to work out; you had a couple of drinks; you have to get up early; there's a great program you've just got to catch on TV; or, maybe, you've got some last minute work to catch up on. No matter what your reason, it's just an excuse.

If you exercise every day at the same time, your body and mind will get accustomed to it and will begin to crave it. If you exercise at 4:00 P.M. every day, for example, your body will begin to prepare itself for that hour. You'll feel eager as the time approaches, restless and itchy if you miss your exercise session. In other words, you'll be hooked. And it's the best addiction you'll ever have.

The Right Place

Finding the right place to exercise is as important as finding the right time. A big part of acquiring discipline is making things easy for yourself. Eliminate distractions and find yourself a place that's conducive to exercise. If you try to do your exercise in the middle of the living room when all the kids are watching cartoons, or if you're expecting a long-distance conference call any second, you'll never make it past the warm-up.

Why do you think most gurus meditate in remote mountain caves? Because they tried keeping their sanity in the big city, and after a while, they realized they'd better find a peaceful place to contemplate. If you're going to have any chance of reaching a physical nirvana through exercise, you've got to find yourself a little place to yourself where no one can annoy you—not the kids, not the boss, not your brother calling collect from Kansas City. Take the phone off the hook —this is your time to exercise!

Groups and Classes

An excellent way to help you stick with your workout is to find an exercise companion, or join a group or class. Working out with a friend at a set time a few days a week gives you the advantage of companionship and encouragement. This interdependence may keep you going when you feel like quitting. And it's a lot more difficult to skip your workout when you know your friend will be calling. Getting going each day is always the toughest part. But once you begin, you almost immediately lose that sluggish feeling that made you feel like skipping your workout.

A group exercise program adds another dimension to a workout. The morale and camaraderie of twenty or thirty people all exercising together is a valuable inducement to stay with your workout. The charged atmosphere in a room of people who feel good about what they're doing can motivate you. Not only is your body beginning to feel better, but the fun of a group session lifts the sagging spirits as well.

A further advantage of a class or group exercise is that you know if you're doing the exercise correctly. Researchers have found that people who exercise correctly—that is, with the proper technique so they avoid injury and get the most out of their workout—tend to stick with an exercise program nearly three times as often as people who don't. It's very hard to know, even when you're facing a mirror, if you're doing a movement correctly. Exercise companions, however, can see if you're exercising the right way and correct you when you're not. A skilled and knowledgeable instructor, of course, is invaluable in keeping you interested and planning the best workout for you.

One other thing: research shows that your chances of sticking with a program are greatly enhanced if your wife approves of and encourages you. If your wife has not yet begun an aerobics program of her own, bring her along to your workouts. Get her involved, and you'll probably find it very hard not to exercise regularly.

What to Look for in a Class

It's very important to find the right class or group to join. The personality of the instructor is the first consideration. If you feel uncomfortable with him, the class will not be much fun. Does he smile? Does he make eye contact with the participants? Does he make you feel like you're part of the group? So many instructors get up in front of the class, with their muscles, their tan, and their expensive exercise outfit, and act as if they're on stage. They make sure you know that they are the instructors and you're the pupil. Unless the instructor appeals to you as a person, try another group.

Another thing about instructors: if your instructor stays too long on each individual exercise (and anything over thirty to forty seconds is excessive), if he constantly harangues the participants to "push until it hurts," you'll be much better off in another class.

The length of the class is also very important. Some programs are too short, but usually exercise classes run too long. I participated in a class in Fiji that was two hours long! At the end of the class, I was exhausted and half of the group had dropped out. A class that runs too long is boring and invites injury. But beyond that, a program that eats up too much of your time is impractical.

When you pick a group, ask yourself if it will fit into your schedule. Not only should it run about forty-five minutes, but it should also start on time and *finish* on time. If you've got an instructor who regularly strolls in fifteen minutes late, find another class. A large part of the reason I stayed with my class in the beginning was that I knew I'd be through at six-thirty promptly. I had a very busy schedule at the time, but I knew I could afford to exercise if the time was well budgeted. If the class goes on too long, you'll feel pressed for time, and you'll neither enjoy nor stick with it.

Make It Fun!

If an aerobics program isn't fun, you won't stay with it. Part of the reward of exercise must be the pleasure of the exercise itself. Even though our ultimate purpose may be to get in shape, avoid heart disease, and achieve general health and well-being, our bodies respond to sensuous activity—the feeling of grace and rhythm associated with anything athletic. We instinctively respond to the fresh air and freedom of running outdoors—of releasing ourselves from the confinement of office work. We have an innate need to counteract the bad effects of inactivity. In the end, we exercise because it makes us feel good. The human body is built to exercise just as an airplane is built to fly.

Unfortunately, most of us have such bad memories of high school calisthenics run by some drill-sergeant football coach that we cringe at the mere mention of exercise. But it doesn't have to be that way. Exercise can be fun.

First of all, don't make your workout into a boot camp. Don't be too hard on yourself. Try never to miss a workout session; but if you do, so what? Today is the best day I can think of to start all over again. Unfortunately, many people quit their workout permanently after they've missed once or twice because they feel they just don't have the will power to succeed. Don't let yourself be defeated by your defeatist attitude. You're out of shape and you've been out of shape for twenty years—but you can turn it all around simply by going out there again today and exercising.

Don't make exercising drudgery. Start slowly and when you feel exhausted, pull back a little. If you don't feel well, don't try so hard. Make your workout enjoyable. Your body will crave exercise just as strongly as it craves chocolate cake if you give it a chance to taste the delights of exercise—and the fun of it.

Tips for the Businessman and Traveler

The pilots of the Eastern Airlines flight to New York suddenly felt a steady, rhythmic thumping sound coming through the floor of the cockpit. They checked out all the instruments and everything was fine, but the thumping continued. Since they were only a short distance from New York, they decided not to call for an emergency landing. Instead, they radioed ahead for the emergency vehicles to be ready.

Finally, as they were nearing JFK airport, a flight attendant noticed that the thumping seemed to be coming from the forward lavatory. And that's when he discovered a business executive, in shorts, finishing his twenty-minute jog-in-place. Nothing was going to stop him from doing his workout.

Many frequent travelers are very serious about maintaining their exercise programs. And the travel industry is catching on to the idea that fitness is important to its customers. Many hotels are now adding health clubs to their facilities for guests. They offer everything from exercise mats for your room to fully equipped gymnasiums with free aerobics classes.

More than two thousand hotels in the United States now offer fitness facilities and programs. The Marriott chain, in fact, has fitness facilities in 60 percent of its properties. The Houstonian in Houston, Texas, billed as "the country's most comprehensive health and fitness complex," staffs twenty-six full-time health and fitness professionals. Its facilities include racquetball and tennis courts, a dance studio, exercise rooms, indoor and outdoor jogging tracks, whirlpools, saunas, and an Olympic-size swimming pool.

The list of hotels that offer special fitness packages and amenities includes Hyatt, Vista-International, Stouffer Hotels, Best Western, and the Marriotts. Cruise ships such as the *Norwegian Carribean* lines, *Queen Elizabeth 2,* and *The Nieuw Amsterdam* also offer a full range of fitness programs. And these are just a small sampling of the places that now cater to the traveling man who wants to stay in shape.

But if you want to keep fit, you don't need to go to a hotel with a gym or a resort with a fancy price tag. You can do your workout with

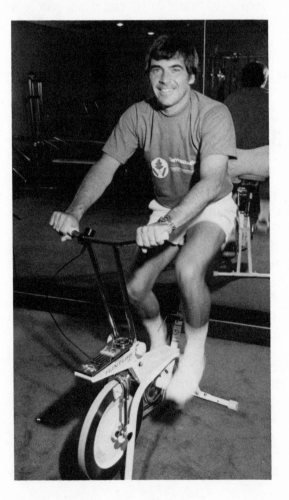

A very good alternative for an aerobic workout is the stationary bicycle. If you ride for a long enough time at a fast enough pace, you'll derive the same benefit. Unfortunately, even if you have access to a bike, you'll still be out of luck when you're traveling. Therefore, an exercise bike should only be a supplement to your regular aerobic workout.

only a small cassette recorder and a cassette of recorded music. If you don't have tennis shoes with you, you can do it barefooted. If you didn't bring your gym shorts, do it in your underwear. That's the beauty of the Aerobic Workout for Men. You can do it almost anywhere, at almost any time.

There are no excuses for not exercising while you're traveling. I've spent three hundred days a year in hotels for the last twenty years. And *nothing* stops me from doing my workout. I used to be self-conscious about stretching and exercising in public, but now I do my workout wherever I find a comfortable place—in a park, in an office, or in a hotel lobby waiting for my room to be prepared.

I have found that the general public is a lot more enlightened these days about fitness. They don't stare at you when they see you working out in a public place. More often they admire a man who takes care of himself. Many of them wish they had the initiative to exercise regularly themselves. And who knows? Seeing you just might be the inspiration they need to get in shape.

Don't fall back on the excuse that you don't have time to exercise. Everybody can find twenty spare minutes to exercise in their hotel rooms. Sure, we're all tired after a long trip, but a good workout will relieve the tension of travel. You'll feel a lot better when you're done, and that overtired feeling will have vanished.

Also, the restless fatigue that often keeps a traveler from sleeping will dissolve if you exercise after you arrive. You'll be ready for a good night's sleep—a rare commodity when you're on the road, in a strange bed, in a different time zone. Next time, instead of drinking too many cocktails to help you fall asleep, just take out your cassette recorder and start your workout.

Finally, a word about "jet lag." I have averaged one and a quarter million air miles a year for nearly twenty years now, and I've found a very simple formula for avoiding jet lag.

1. Don't eat on the plane. Just drink juices or water. Do not drink coffee, tea, or alcohol! They dehydrate you.
2. On a long flight, get up every so often and take a walk around the cabin.
3. Set your watch ahead to the time zone of your destination, so that psychologically you've already begun to adjust. If you try to sleep and eat according to your old time schedule, your body will never feel comfortable in the new time zone.

I've given these simple directions for avoiding jet lag to literally thousands of people over the years and I've found that it works most of the time.

CHAPTER 14

WHAT GOES IN, MUST COME OFF: THE IMPORTANCE OF DIET

Studies have shown that many affluent Americans suffer from malnutrition. At the same time, 40 percent of all Americans are obese. We are overfed but undernourished because our eating habits do not supply us with the proper nutrients. Statistics show that we prefer highly processed foods that are loaded with sugar, fat, salt, and chemicals—but few nutrients. Throw in our addictions to alcohol, tobacco, and other drugs, from sleeping pills to marijuana, and it's obvious that if we're going to get fit, we've got to educate ourselves about the things we put into our bodies.

You can exercise better and more efficiently if you're running on the proper fuel. That's why, for example, distance runners usually eat a lot of complex carbohydrates. A good exercise program should go hand-in-hand with a sensible, healthy approach to diet.

Some Things You Should Know about Food

Anyone interested in his health should know at least some basic facts about nutrition. Remember, the food you eat is utilized as fuel, which gives you the energy to exercise.

Protein

If you're the average American, you're probably getting at least three times the protein you need, and about seventy times more protein than the average Asian consumes! And if you consume protein drinks one, two, or three times a day, you're probably drowning yourself in the stuff.

Excess protein poisons your system by dumping into it too much uric acid, waste nitrogen, and other toxic substances that overwork your kidneys and liver. Protein has also been found to drastically stimulate aging, which explains why the Masai, an African tribe whose diet is almost exclusively meat, show signs of advanced age in their late twenties. Heavy meat-eating societies, such as the Eskimos, the Greenlanders, the Russian Kirghiz, and the Masai have a life expectancy of about thirty to forty years.

Nutrients are only safe or useful to the body up to a certain point. Because of our fears and our ignorance, we are destroying our bodies by giving them nutrients well beyond their needs.

But don't misunderstand me—protein is vitally important to your body. It is a part of every living cell and is found in every organism, from the amoeba to the whale. In fact, the only substance more plentiful than protein in the body is water. We are 20 percent protein by weight.

Only protein contains nitrogen, sulfur, and phosphorous—substances essential to life. Muscles, bones, and skin are made mostly of protein. And protein is needed to replace tissues that are continually breaking down and growing, such as hair and nails. It is also crucial during such periods of growth as childhood and pregnancy.

Protein is essential to major metabolic functions, such as heat regulation and water balance. The bloated stomach commonly seen on starving children, for example, is caused by fluid allowed to accumulate in the interstitial spaces between the cells and is a direct result of protein deficiency. A lack of protein in the system can also cause mental and physical retardation, anemia, excessive weight loss, irritability, and reduced natural immunities.

As protein from your diet is digested, it breaks down into the organic acids called amino acids. Though it takes from a couple of days to seven years to deplete the body's reserves of other required nutrients, amino acid reserves are depleted in a few hours. Since cells must be constantly repaired and replaced (red blood cells have a life span of only about 120 days and the lining of the small intestine is renewed every day or two), an adequate supply of protein must be maintained.

How much protein do we need? Technically speaking, we need enough to keep our bodies in a "positive nitrogen balance," which means that there is more protein in the body than is being used. Since protein is made up mostly of nitrogen, if you measure the amount of nitrogen going in and out of the body, you can figure your nitrogen balance. If you are in a negative nitrogen balance, then you are losing protein from your muscles and you've got a problem.

Just as serious a problem is an excess positive nitrogen balance. If you get more than about 16 percent protein in your diet, you'll have a negative mineral balance. The reason is that high amounts of protein set up an acid condition, and only calcium leached from the bones can neutralize this effect. The brittle bones of the aged are often attributed to a lack of milk in their diets. But it is actually a protein-saturated diet throughout their lives that leaches calcium from their systems and causes this problem.

The average American consumes at least 20 percent of his or her diet in proteins, yet studies have shown that adults who ate only white rice (6 percent protein) as their main protein source maintained a positive nitrogen balance. I don't recommend eating only white rice, or even keeping your protein intake to 6 percent. But a sensible level, suggested by the World Health Organization, is between 10 and 15 percent.

If you know how many calories you should consume daily to maintain a sensible weight for your height, age, and activity level, it is simple to compute your protein needs. Simply multiply your calorie intake by 10 percent for your minimum protein requirement.

There are several factors, however, that do vary protein requirements. There is evidence that stress can cause protein deficiency. Fear or prolonged anxiety increases the levels of adrenaline in the system, and this burns up protein. Loss of sleep, jet lag, fever, infection, surgery, and any other occurrences that upset normal metabolic patterns can also deplete protein supplies up to one-third over the normal rate. But don't go overboard. If you're taking in over 15 percent of your calories in protein on a regular basis, you're doing yourself more harm than good.

Carbohydrates and Sugar

Carbohydrates are usually divided into starches and sugars. They are made up of carbon, oxygen, and hydrogen, and are found in fruits, vegetables, grains, nuts, seeds, and the roots and cellulose of plants.

Carbohydrates are the body's main fuel for exercise, and they are much more efficient than fats or proteins as muscular fuel. An abundant supply of carbohydrates saves the proteins in your system for their job of body and cell maintenance.

Carbohydrates must be converted into glucose before they can be utilized by your body. Glucose is one of the simple sugars, and it transports its fuels through the bloodstream. Starches are made up of complex chains of glucose and are, therefore, easily broken down during the digestive processes to form glucose for energy.

On the other hand, the carbohydrates in sugar and bleached and processed flours are devoid of nutrients. Although these foods satisfy your appetite, they use up calories that could have been better spent on foods that supply vitamins and minerals. Whole grains and legumes, for instance, supply the B vitamins that the body needs to burn glucose as fuel; but, even more important, the proteins, fats, and roughage found in complex carbohydrates slow down the digestion of glucose and allow sugars to burn up slowly and steadily. That's the reason why, when you eat a plate of spaghetti, for example, you don't feel the sudden rush and subsequent letdown that usually follows a chocolate bar or doughnuts and coffee.

Carbohydrates from unprocessed whole grains and legumes, as well as raw fruits and vegetables, can satisfy both your appetite and your nutritional needs. That's why I stress that a great proportion of your diet should consist of the complex carbohydrates.

The popular notion that you should stay away from carbohydrates because they're fattening is a myth. They are fattening only if you consume too many total calories. Otherwise, they are no more fattening than an equivalent number of calories of fat or protein.

The real culprits in the carbohydrate family are those that are highly refined—empty-calorie foods such as sugar, white flour, and alcohol. These processed carbohydrates fill you up with calories but have almost no nutrients. Also, because they burn up so quickly, they cause drastic and rapid fluctuations in your blood-sugar level.

The emphasis on processed carbohydrates in this country has caused a shift in our diets from mostly starch to mostly sugar. Seventy-five years ago, 55 percent of our carbohydrate intake was starch. Today, starch accounts for 37 percent. Sugars now account for nearly 40 percent of our carbohydrate consumption—twice the amount we ate in 1920. Today, the average American consumes two pounds of sugar a week, 125 pounds a year (150 pounds a year for children), from hundreds of sources—table sugar, soft drinks, desserts, breads, sauces, and canned goods.

This emphasis on sugar has created massive physiological problems, including increased blood pressure, hypoglycemia, diabetes, embolism, and heart disease. Cirrhosis of the liver has been found in teenagers who consume too many soft drinks.

Stay away from refined sugar (even brown and raw sugar) and any processed foods that contain it. They are all basically sucrose, which lowers the blood sugar and triggers abnormal insulin reactions. Also, honey, though superior to any other sweetener, is still a sugar and, like all sugars, promotes dental cavities, obesity, and emotional and physical ups and downs.

Carbohydrates or Protein for Energy?

Many athletes, in an effort to increase muscle bulk and their strength, go on high-protein diets. This is a mistake for two reasons: first, a balanced diet supplies far more protein than you need for even the most demanding sport; and second, protein is the least efficient energy source. The digestion of excess protein actually requires about five times as much energy as the digestion of carbohydrates or fats. The amino acids that make up protein must be converted into carbohydrates and go through additional reactions before they can be utilized for energy. The by-products of this metabolism must then be eliminated by the kidneys.

A further drawback to excess protein consumption for an athlete is the dehydrating effects of a high-protein regimen, because the body demands much larger amounts of water to eliminate protein by-products than carbohydrate by-products. In general, then, proteins are inefficient sources of energy and are used for energy by the body only when the more efficient sources, carbohydrates and fats, are not available.

Most sports nutritionists say that if you plan to train seriously for competition, your carbohydrate consumption should exceed more than half your diet.

One important point that you should be aware of, however, is that carbohydrates cannot be stored in any significant amount in the body. In fact, only enough for about twelve hours of very light activity can be stored. Heavy exercise can deplete your carbohydrate stores in a couple of hours. So instead of eating large meals two or three times a day, eat small carbohydrate-packed meals and snacks throughout the day.

Fats and Cholesterol

Fat is just as important to your diet as protein. Fat is used for energy reserves so that your protein supply will not be used as fuel. Fat pads the internal organs from injury and is vital in both the production of body heat and as an insulator to preserve that heat. It is also required for the absorption of the fat-soluble vitamins A, D, E, and K.

On the other hand, too much fat can kill you. Excess fatty deposits significantly impair the cleansing action of the liver and kidneys and raise cholesterol to dangerous levels. Most important of all, excessive fat in the diet is closely linked to heart disease. The American Heart Association specifically recommends limiting the cholesterol in your diet to reduce the risk of heart disease.

You should, however, be aware of the importance of polyunsaturated fats.

Dietary fats are divided into two major groups, depending on how many hydrogen atoms are capable of being bonded to their carbon chains. If fats are saturated with all the hydrogen they can hold, they are called saturated fats. If they are unsaturated because their double bonds remain available for more hydrogen, they are usually called polyunsaturated.

In general, saturated fats, such as butter and lard, are solid at room temperature, whereas unsaturated fats, such as most vegetable oils, are liquid at room temperature. Animal fats are highly saturated, and vegetable and fish oils are highly unsaturated (except for coconut, palm, and olive oil).

Food manufacturers, in an effort to increase profits, have advertised polyunsaturated fats as a panacea for coronary heart disease. This is simply not true. Although polyunsaturated fats are more easily digested, some studies have shown that a diet loaded with them can cause hair loss, diarrhea, and liver dysfunction. Polyunsaturates also cause a blood condition known as "sludging," which reduces the blood flow, especially in the lungs. It is most dangerous for people with such diseases as emphysema and asthma and for those who live in areas with highly polluted air.

Although polyunsaturates contain no cholesterol, it is fat, as well as cholesterol, that affects the serum cholesterol—the cholesterol in the blood.

About 40 to 45 percent of the average American's caloric intake consists of fats—over one hundred pounds per year for every adult. This is well over recommended limits or nutritional requirements. Actually, a well-balanced diet contains no more than about 15 percent of its calories in fats of all types.

Fat is a concentrated source of calories and energy. There is twice as much energy by weight in fats as in proteins and carbohydrates. Fat is present in all meats, as well as in breads, cakes, and cookies. And those sources alone will supply you with all the dietary fat you need. But the greatest proportion of your fat intake comes from such foods as gravies, ice cream, salad dressings, and fried foods. All these extra fats are choking your system with cholesterol and fatty tissue.

Fiber

The indigestible part of plants, known as roughage or fiber, adds nothing of nutritive value to your diet but can eliminate constipation and many accompanying ills. The fiber in your food helps push the waste products through your system more rapidly, which means these bacteria-laden substances have less time to putrefy in your body. Putrefaction of waste matter is considered by many experts to be a major contributor to illness—lowering the effectiveness of your body's immune system and fostering disease. Studies have shown that people who consume only small amounts of fiber suffer high rates of cancer of the colon. The best sources of fiber are whole-grain cereals, nuts, and raw fruits and vegetables.

Water

Seventy percent of a man's body weight is water, and water is vital for every bodily function from carrying nutrients along the bloodstream to thinking. It takes nearly a gallon and a half of water every day just to replace the water the body loses by breathing, sweating, and elimination.

During weight loss the intake of water is doubly important since fat is being expelled from the body, taking water with it. If you overexercise or follow a crash diet in which rapid weight loss occurs, the loss of water can be critical. In fact, most of the weight lost through radical dieting is mostly due to the loss of water, which explains why most of the weight comes back so quickly. Whenever you exercise or diet, always drink at least two or three extra glasses of water a day.

Drink a glass of water a half an hour before and, of course, shortly after you work out. Also, the hotter the day, the more water you should drink before and after you exercise.

Variety and Balance:
The Keys to a Healthy Diet

The key to a sane, healthy, and enjoyable approach to eating is to consume a varied and balanced diet. Choose a wide selection of foods from the four basic food groups listed on page 137 and never get in the rut of eating the same thing day in and day out.

Also, avoid the trap of trying to meticulously plot out your nutritional needs down to the exact milligram. Calculating how many calories of this protein food and that mineral source isn't necessary. You don't have to buy every vitamin supplement on the shelf to ensure that you've got all possible nutritional angles covered. Be sensible. The best way to guarantee that you get sufficient quantities of all necessary trace minerals and vitamins, and all the other nutrients that make up a sound diet, is simply to eat a wide range of different foods.

The Four Basic Food Groups

The Protein Group: Cheeses and Beans *

Included in this group are beans and cheeses of all kinds.

Grains, Legumes, Nuts, and Seeds

Grains: some examples are rice, bread, oats, pasta, cereal, wheat germ, and flour.

Legumes: some examples are chick peas (garbanzo beans), pinto beans, kidney beans, peanuts, lentils, soybeans, and split peas.

Nuts and seeds: some examples are almonds, cashews, pecans, pistachios, pumpkin seeds, sesame seeds, sunflower seeds, and walnuts.

Fruits and Vegetables

Included in this group are fresh, wholesome vegetables and fruits and fruit juices of all varieties.

Dairy Products

Included in this group are milk, cheese, yogurt, cottage cheese, ricotta, kefir, sour cream, and cream.

Hints for a Healthy Diet

Eating a sensible, varied diet while avoiding "empty" calories and excessive sugar and saturated fats should keep your body working, and playing, at its best. Here are a few hints, however, that may help:

Eat as Many Unprocessed Foods as Possible

Avoid processed or canned foods—you never know what's in them. If you do buy food that is packaged, make sure you read the label. Check for additives such as chemical coloring, flavoring, preservatives, and sugar.

* Note since I am a lacto-vegetarian I cannot recommend the eating of meats, poultry, fish, and eggs, which would ordinarily be included in this group.

Eat Whole-Wheat and Whole-Grain Breads and Cereals

Most of the food value has been removed from "enriched" white flour and only about one-sixth of it has been replaced. Why take in empty calories, calories with no nutritional value?

Avoid Added Sugar

Refined white sugar and foods "enriched" with it act destructively on the body, leeching it of vitamins and minerals. Brown sugar is just white sugar covered with molasses. A little honey in recipes isn't bad, but sugar is sugar. If possible, reeducate your tastes.

Swear Off Junk Foods and Beverages

Junk food is anything that contains little or no essential nutrients but is filled with calories that crowd out other nutritionally rich foods. It might not be easy to give them up at first, but reading what's actually in those "fabricated foods" should strengthen your resolve.

Think twice before buying convenience foods.

Limit Your Intake of Salt

Most of us take in more salt than we need just by eating processed foods and snack foods. But when we add salt to cooked meals at the table, we consume up to ten times the amount of salt that we need. Salt is essential to human life. Our body water and our blood are maintained at a precise salinity, and it's these salt levels that allow us to keep body moisture stable. Excessive salt in the diet, however, can lead to liver and kidney disease and high blood pressure.

If you refrain from salting your food, it will not be long before your taste for salt diminishes and you find out what the food you eat really tastes like. Next time you eat, taste your food before you add salt. You might like it better that way.

Beware of Crash Diets

The rapid weight loss that occurs due to a crash or starvation diet is unhealthy and even dangerous. When you restrict your intake of food to one thousand calories a day or less, the body can lose its energy, endurance, muscle tone, and resistance to disease. Also, diets based on only one food, such as grapefruit or brown rice or liquid protein mixes, are nutritionally inadequate and can lead to illness.

Here are some common-sense guides to follow when dieting:

1. Be realistic about weight loss. If you lose more than one or two pounds per week, your diet is probably not safe.

2. Reduce your intake of calories but continue to eat a balanced diet selected from the four basic food groups.
3. Exercise to firm up muscles and lose weight. A well-conditioned person burns more calories even while sleeping than someone who's out of shape.

Vegetarianism—Something to Think About

One day in 1971, when I was resting between tennis tournaments, I was throwing a Frisbee around on the beach in Waikiki with a bunch of my friends and accidentally hit a man on the head with it. I went over to apologize and it turned out he was a doctor and was in town attending a medical symposium on diets. The theme of the symposium was that meat was the worst thing you could put in your body. I remember thinking I wanted to get back to the Frisbee, but I felt obliged to sit there and listen to the doctor because I had hit him on the head. He started drawing charts in the sand and telling me that an athlete should not eat meat six months before an event. Finally, he persuaded me to come to the symposium.

I went with seven of my friends—five men and two women. We showed up at the Hilton Hawaiian Village Convention Hall, where there were three hundred doctors in suits and ties. We looked like beach bums—barefooted, wearing bathing suits, and hauling surfboards. We sat in the back by the door, with the surfboards propped up against the wall, so we could escape unnoticed. We'd all made a deal that as soon as it got boring we'd head back to the beach. We expected to stay no more than five minutes or so.

Five hours later, after dozens of speakers and demonstrations and statistics and studies and tests, after the very last speaker, we finally left. I gave up meat that day, and I have not touched it, or fish, poultry, and eggs, since. That's how convinced I was.

But the real test came when I went to Lloyd Percival's Fitness Center in Toronto, Canada. Percival tested all of the top athletes in the country. From 1967 to 1969, when I was a meat eater, I was rated between number fifty and sixty. The year I stopped eating meat I really wanted to do well in the test, because by then I'd become a "vegetarian fugitive." (I refused to discuss my eating habits or go out to dinner with anyone because I was embarrassed to be a vegetarian. My parents thought I was crazy, and all the players on the circuit constantly ribbed me.)

To do well on the fitness test, I had to at least score in the top sixty again. But things were not looking good for me. The day before the test, I played in the finals of a tournament in St. Petersburg, Florida. Billie Jean King and Chris Evert were in the women's finals right before me, and they had a long match. Then I got into a long match myself and missed my plane for Toronto. I got a late plane to Cleveland and ended up sleeping on a bench at the Hopkins Airport in Cleveland so I could catch the 7:00 A.M. flight to Toronto. When I got off the plane in Toronto I went right to the Fitness Center, and I felt the way anyone would feel after sleeping on a bench in an airport—totally exhausted.

The testing procedure lasted for fourteen hours. About halfway through it, a doctor burst into my room and screamed, "What have you been doing? You've improved 20 percent in this area and 50 percent in that area and 38 percent in this area." After a year of being a vegetarian fugitive, the doctor's figures proved that I had been right all along.

I hadn't been doing any special training, I didn't run, I'd just been playing my regular tournament schedule; plus, I was traveling a lot, which puts a great strain on the body. But the testing showed that I was the fittest athlete of all those being tested.

Vegetarianism changed my life, made me healthier, happier, and a better tennis player, with more energy and stamina and a better mental outlook. But it also gave me insights that opened up a whole new way of thinking for me.

If vegetarianism seems extreme, then at least, for the health of your body, cut down on your intake of meat. Or, if you want to know more about vegetarianism, you can read my book *Peter Burwash's Vegetarian Primer*. Available through Peter Burwash International, 2203 Timberloch Place, Suite 126, Woodlands, Texas, 77386. $14.95, plus $1.00 for shipping.

Cigarettes, Alcohol, and Coffee

"The Surgeon General has determined that cigarette smoking is hazardous to your health." Need I say more? Apparently, I must, because every year one million people take up smoking as a regular habit, even though it's common knowledge that it can kill you. Smokers develop atherosclerosis and degeneration of the heart muscle. The lungs collect tar, which leads to emphysema and lung cancer. In short, cigarette smoking is probably the worst health habit a person can develop —especially if you want to get in shape.

Alcohol is another drug to be avoided. It's high in empty calories that provide the body with almost no nourishment. In addition to speeding up the process of aging, alcohol can cause gastrointestinal problems by irritating the lining of the stomach and intestines. Prolonged use of alcohol can cause cirrhosis of the liver and lead to brain and nerve damage. If you drink a lot, it's also much harder to stick with your workout. Alcohol creates a lethargic feeling in the body, which persists for days and can affect your desire to exercise.

The use of coffee, tea, soft drinks, and other beverages that contain caffeine can cause insomnia, diarrhea, gastritis, heart palpitations, and nervous disorders of all types. Also, caffeine addiction can seriously affect exercise. The artificial high you get from caffeine drinks will distort heart response and can make you feel tired when you're not and elated when you should feel tired.

Because caffeine withdrawal can be severe, causing headaches and flulike symptoms, it's probably best to gradually reduce your intake of caffeine. But no matter how you do it, by all means, give up caffeine.

CHAPTER 15

INJURIES: PREVENTION AND CURE

Some Common-Sense Tips

Don't Overexercise!

The first rule of injury prevention is *don't overdo it!* Set realistic goals for yourself and "listen" to your body for signs of pain, weakness, and fatigue.

Avoid pushing yourself too hard, especially in the beginning. Overdoing it the first few weeks after starting a regular exercise program is probably the major cause of exercise-related injuries. Take it slow and easy in the beginning, monitor your heart rate closely, and only do as much as you can.

Probably the major offender of the "don't overdo it" rule is the ex-athlete. It's hard for him to understand that an exercise program is not a competition. He thinks he can regain his past glory overnight. But instead, he inevitably pulls a muscle or a tendon or injures himself in some other way.

Remember, there's always someone out there who can swim faster, run farther, and lift more weight than you. The aerobics program described in this book is designed to fit your personal needs. If you exercise according to these guidelines, you will be fit, trim, and healthy.

There are some signs that will warn you if you are overexercising:

1. If at any time during your exercise you feel dizzy, lightheaded, nauseous, breathless or a pain or tightness in your chest, stop exercising immediately.

2. If you are still short of breath ten minutes after you stopped exercising, you're overdoing it. Or if your pulse rate is over 120 five minutes later, or over 100 ten minutes later, you're probably exercising too hard.
3. General fatigue indicates that you're pushing yourself too hard. If you feel tired all day after working out, you have trouble sleeping because you're exhausted, or your muscles are constantly sore, cut back on your exercise schedule. Take a day off.
4. You should be able to carry on a normal conversation while exercising aerobically. If you're gasping for breath and can barely push out a few words as you exercise, you're working out too strenuously.

Don't Exercise When You're Sick

When your health is in any way impaired, *do not exercise!* If you have a cold, minor infection, or a muscle or tendon injury, take a few days off. If you have a fever, wait at least one day *after* your temperature returns to normal before you exercise.

Strenuous exercise can delay recovery and even aggravate illness and injury. Rest one day for every day you were sick and resume exercise gradually. Start with light exercise and monitor your heart rate closely.

Beware of Extreme Climatic Conditions

Avoid exercising in extremes of heat, cold, and humidity, unless you are in top physical condition or have become acclimated to the elements. Any time the mercury moves below forty-five degrees or above eighty-five degrees, or the humidity is more than 60 percent, beware.

Heat exhaustion and heat stroke are the two most common conditions people suffer while exercising in hot weather.

The symptoms of heat exhaustion are thirst, weakness, fatigue, nausea, and disorientation. To treat it, move the victim to a cool place and have him drink cool water. Toweling the face, arms, legs, and stomach with a cool, damp cloth also helps.

Heat stroke is very serious and can be fatal. The victim may pass out and his body temperature can climb above 102 degrees. If he is conscious, headaches, disorientation, dizziness, and shock may occur. To administer first aid, apply ice water to his entire body. Get him to a hospital immediately.

There are measures you can take to avoid heat-related problems. In hot weather, wear light clothing and give your body time to adjust to the heat. When you go on vacation and the temperature is much hotter than you are used to, avoid the temptation to run around in the hot sun. Hold back for a few days. Also, be aware that so-called "sports beverages" are often heavily salted and sweetened. Cool water is more effective in preventing and treating heat-related injuries.

Unless the temperature is below zero, a physically fit person does not usually have to worry about cold weather. But if you're out of shape, you should avoid all extremes—not only exercising too long or hard, but also in weather that's too cold.

Inhaling ice cold air can cause a sudden cooling in the neck and chest, which could trigger vasoconstriction of the heart muscles. This reduces the oxygen flow to the heart and can cause a heart attack. If you feel any tightness or pain in the chest while working out in cold weather, stop exercising immediately.

When exercising in cold weather, wear several layers of warm, dry clothing. This enables air to circulate between the clothes, insulating and aiding evaporation of sweat. Wear warm gloves. And wear a hat. More than half of our body heat is lost through the scalp. Adequate head covering will help keep your entire body warm.

Be careful when exercising at altitudes more than two thousand feet higher than where you live. The thinner air at higher altitudes reduces your intake of oxygen and makes the lungs and heart work harder.

Questionable Exercise Practices

Dangerous Exercises

Just about any exercise can be harmful if done incorrectly. But there are a lot of exercises still included in many fitness programs that are contrary to safe fitness standards. Exercises such as straight-legged situps, toe touches, back arches, and deep knee bends should be strictly avoided.

The straight-legged situp is supposed to strengthen the stomach muscles. But most of the work is actually done by the muscles that run from the lower back to the thighs. This exercise can cause serious hypertension of the lower back and crippling back problems.

Toe touches can overstress the ligaments of the knees and the lower back and cause serious spinal disc complications. If you must bounce to touch your toes, the negative effects of toe touches are compounded.

Deep knee bends should be strictly avoided. Squatting so low that the heels touch the buttocks excessively stretches the ligaments and exposes the knee to injury.

Back arches, in which the back is hyperextended, can permanently weaken the ligaments of the vertebrae. They also increase the forward curve of the spine, which can cause "sway back."

Saunas, Steambaths, and Rubber Sweatsuits

Saunas, steambaths, and rubber sweatsuits all have one thing in common: they make you sweat. Since water weighs a lot (over a pound per pint), you can lose ten pounds or more during an hour of exercise. But sweating is a dangerous and completely ineffective way of losing weight. Rapid water loss causes dehydration and an imbalance of the body's chemicals. And you immediately regain any weight lost this way as soon as you drink water. Fat is not burned by overheating the body artificially through saunas, steambaths, and sweatsuits. Also, heat exhaustion can follow a rapid water loss, especially in hot weather.

The Myth of Salt Tablets

Never take salt tablets. Salt will prevent muscle cramps, but the damage that a concentrated tablet can do to your stomach, digestive tract, and blood pressure is not worth the risk. Excessive salt in your system will draw the fluids out of your cells and into your digestive tract, so that the salt can be diluted and then expelled from the body. But this can leave you dehydrated, and dehydration can lead to cramps —which is what salt tablets are supposed to prevent.

If you are prone to cramping, you can increase your intake of salt by adding salt to your food at the table. But be careful: the negative effects of salt, like high blood pressure (which can bring on heart, liver, and kidney failure), often outweigh the positive effects.

If you're bothered by cramps, stretch your entire body for fifteen or twenty minutes every day to loosen your muscles.

Treating Common Exercise Injuries

Probably the biggest obstacle to a successful fitness program is an injury. Just when it seems you finally have the motivation and discipline to stay with your workout, an injury prevents you from exercising.

There are some very effective precautions you can follow to prevent most of the injuries commonly suffered by participants in a conditioning program. And if you are injured, there are some well-tested procedures that will help you recover as quickly as possible.

I have not tried to explain or offer a treatment for every injury suffered by an athlete, but just the most common ones. These injuries usually fall into three categories: muscle problems, tendon and joint problems, and back problems.

General First Aid

When you're injured, the initial treatment is crucial. The first aid you administer minutes after an injury occurs can determine how extensive the injury will be and how long it will take to heal.

There is a simple way to remember what to do immediately after you suffer an injury to a muscle, tendon, ligament, bone, or joint. Just remember R.I.C.E.—which stands for "rest, ice, compression, and elevation."

Rest

As soon as you feel any pain, stop exercising. Rest for at least one day. This limits the chances of further injury and bleeding. It also helps remove excess fluids from the area. When the pain subsides completely, you can begin exercising the affected area—but very slowly.

Ice

Apply ice packs to the injured area to reduce the pain and swelling. But do not apply ice directly to your skin. Use a cloth or apply oil to the area for protection against the extreme cold.

Compression

Wrap an elastic compression bandage firmly over the ice pack. Do not wrap it so tightly, however, that you cut off circulation. Leave the bandage on for thirty minutes, then unwrap it for fifteen minutes. Repeat this process for at least three hours.

Elevation

Position the injured area so it is above the level of your heart. If your leg or ankle is injured, lie down with your leg raised above shoulder height. This helps drain fluids from the injured area, which brings down the swelling.

If you follow the R.I.C.E. prescription for the first forty-eight hours following your injury, it can help you reduce the effects of that injury. You should be aware, also, that applying heat or exercising the affected area too soon after an injury can do further damage. Heat in the form of hot water, hot packs, or heating pads should be applied only after the bleeding inside a muscle has stopped. This will usually take at least two or three days.

Muscle Soreness, Cramps, and Pulls

Our muscles enable us to move because they can shorten and then release to exert force with the help of the joints. Since they are elastic, they can stretch to greater lengths and then snap back. A muscle injury typically occurs when the muscle is not strong enough or flexible enough for the task it is trying to perform. This leads to the three main muscle problems: muscle soreness, cramps, and pulls.

Muscle soreness is usually a minor problem brought on by overexercising. Lactic acid causes an irritation in the cells of overworked muscles and stiffness and soreness often follow within eight hours. To prevent muscle soreness, don't overexercise. Progress slowly, building in intensity and duration as your muscles become conditioned.

Also, be sure to warm up properly before you exercise by stretching the muscles thoroughly. And follow your exercise with a gradual cool-down, which should also include a lot of stretching. Avoid dynamic stretching in which you bounce or force the muscle to stretch.

There is no cure for muscle soreness except stretching. You can treat the pain, however, with linament or aspirin.

Muscle cramps are a sustained contraction of the muscle fibers. Cramps can last for a few seconds or for several hours and are very painful. They usually occur when you exercise too hard and too long on a hot day. Resting, drinking plenty of water, and massaging the affected muscles are the best treatments.

Muscle Pulls are actually a tear of the muscle tissue usually caused by a sudden, forceful movement, a misstep or a sudden stop. Insufficient training, overtraining, improper warm-up, and poor flexibility are the primary causes of pulls.

The best ways to prevent them are to warm up properly and to maintain maximum flexibility with a regular and thorough stretching program. Often a long period of exercise is needed to restore strength and flexibility to the injured muscle. During the first twenty-four hours, apply ice packs or immerse the injured area in ice baths. After that, try whirlpool or hot tub treatments for ten minutes and very slow, easy stretching of the affected area.

Tendon and Joint Injuries

Injuries to the tendons and joints can be tricky because it's so difficult to know exactly what is injured. There are so many tendons, cartilages, ligaments, nerves, and blood vessels in the affected areas that the pain and stiffness can be the result of any number of injuries. "Tennis elbow," for example, is a soreness of the muscles along the back of the elbow. "Runner's knee" is inflamed knee cartilage, and "football knee" is stretched-out ligaments of the knee joint.

Heat and cold treatments are the standard procedure for almost all tendon and joint injuries. But swimming can also help, because it mildly exercises the injured area without putting weight or pressure on it.

Tendinitis is an inflammation of a joint caused by tearing or irritation of the surrounding tendons. Tendons can also rupture; you'll be able to hear a telltale popping sound as they separate from the bone. They heal only by growing new tendon filaments, which reattach to the bone.

The intense pain caused by tendinitis often results in a muscular imbalance because the victim will favor the affected area. This can lead to other injuries.

The most common forms of tendinitis are "tennis elbow"; shin splints, which are caused by an inflamed tendon that has become separated from the shin bone; Achilles tendinitis, which affects the tendon directly above the heel; and sprained ankles, the most frequent tendon injury among athletes and nonathletes alike.

The immediate treatment for tendinitis is to stop any strenuous exercise of the affected area. Ice packs and aspirin will help reduce pain and swelling. After the pain subsides, you should begin some slow, easy stretching of the area to relieve muscle tightness. But take care: any strenuous use of the inflamed tendons can lead to chronic tendinitis, which may cause a buildup of scar tissue surrounding the injury. Then surgery may be required.

Also, avoid cortisone shots or other anti-inflammatory drugs, if possible. Although they may stop the pain, they are only masking the symptoms of a serious injury that can become crippling if you continue to exercise while you are still injured.

Ankle sprains are a tearing of the tendons and tissue surrounding the ankle. If the sprain is minor, some swelling and discomfort will occur, but the joint will be stable. If the tendon is completely ripped away from the ankle bone, resulting in severe swelling and pain, the tear may have to be treated surgically.

To treat a minor sprain, keep the ankle elevated above the level of the heart. Ice the affected area immediately, and have a doctor check for a fracture. An elastic compress bandage also helps support the ankle and keeps swelling down. Do not wrap the bandage too tightly, however, since it will act as a tourniquet and actually increase the swelling.

A complete rehabilitation program for a major sprain, which should be supervised by your doctor, includes whirlpool, ice, and heat treatments, and perhaps even ultrasound techniques, which uses high frequency sound waves to stimulate healing.

Knee problems are often caused by a roughening of the surface on the inside of the kneecap, which causes pain when you move the knee. The other common causes of knee problems are overstretching the knee ligaments and inflammation of the knee cartilage, which causes the knee cap to move beyond its normal groove. If it hits a nerve, you get a shot of pain.

Exercising the quadriceps can help prevent and relieve these conditions. Sit on the edge of a table and slowly raise your leg until it's fully extended. Lower it slowly. Repeat ten to fifteen times. After the knee begins to feel better, add a small weight to your foot to help strengthen the muscles and tendons surrounding the knee.

Shin splints are an inflammation of the muscles and tendons surrounding the tibia, resulting in pain or tightness behind the front bone of the lower leg. They are usually caused by overexercising or by exercising on a hard surface such as pavement or a tennis court. But improper footwear can also cause shin splints. If your shoes are old or broken down or not built for vigorous exercise, they can cause you serious injuries.

Shin splints often strike people just starting to exercise again after a long layoff or people who actively engage in two or more sports. Just because you're in condition for tennis does not mean your muscles and tendons are ready for everything. Don't assume that because you jog regularly you're also in shape for aerobics.

Shin splints require rest—perhaps for as long as several weeks. If severe enough, crutches may be necessary. You can also try hot and cold treatments: ten minutes of wet heat, followed by twenty minutes of ice packs. Aspirin will help reduce the pain and swelling.

Stress fractures are not a ligament injury, but they are often confused with shin splints. Therefore, if you have any of the symptoms of shin splints, it might be wise to have your doctor X-ray for a stress fracture. If the injury is detected early and treated, it can heal completely. But often stress fractures are not detected on the initial X-rays and the victim will try to "run through the pain." If you continue to exercise when you have a stress fracture or try to mask the pain with cortisone or other anti-inflammatory drugs, you can cause the bone to fracture completely.

Rest is the best medicine for a stress fracture and the best prevention is to avoid frequent overtraining and running on pavement. Also, proper footwear can aid stability and help cushion the area.

Back Problems

Back injuries have reached epidemic proportions. Over one-third of our adult population suffers from some type of back ailment. Most of those ailments are created or intensified by an overall lack of fitness. Weak stomach and back muscles create tightness, strains and spasms of the lower back, in particular.

The best way to prevent back injury is to follow a regular stretching routine, such as the one I've laid out in the "Workout" section of this book. Stretch the muscles of the back, torso, and stomach. Also, avoid straining the back through weight training, lifting heavy objects such as furniture, and bending from the waist to pick things up off the floor. Try sleeping on your side on a firm mattress, avoid standing or sitting for long periods of time, and apply wet heat to the painful area. If the pain is severe and persists, or radiates down into your leg, see your doctor.

NOTES

1. "National Poll Lists Barriers To Maintenance of Health," *The President's Council on Physical Fitness and Sports Newsletter,* Sept. 1980.
2. "Exploring the Frontiers of Fitness Knowledge," *The Physician and Sportsmedicine,* May 1976, p. 108.
3. "American Lifestyle," *The Michigan Journal for Health, Physical Education, and Recreation,* October 1976, p. 12.
4. J. Mayer, *Overweight: Causes, Cost and Control* (Englewood Cliffs, N.J.: Prentice-Hall, 1968), p. 82.
5. W. B. Kannel, P. Sorlie, and P. McNamara, "The Relation of Physical Activity to Risk of Coronary Heart Disease: The Framingham Study," in O. A. Larsen and R. O. Malborg (eds.), *Coronary Heart Disease and Physical Fitness* (Baltimore, University Park Press, 1971), p. 256.
6. R. S. Paffenbarger, M. E. Laughlim, A. S. Gima, and R. A. Black, "Work Activity of Longshoremen as Related to Death From Coronary Heart Disease and Stroke," *New England Journal of Medicine* 20 (1970): 1109.
7. J. N. Morris, C. Adams, S. P. W. Chave, C. Sirey, and D. J. Sheehan, "Vigorous Exercise in Leisure Time and the Incidence of Coronary Heart Disease," *The Lancet* 285 (1973): 333.
8. Ibid.
9. R. A. Berger, "Effects of Varied Weight Training Programs on Strength," *Research Quarterly* 33 (1962): 175–76.
10. K. H. Cooper, *Aerobics* (New York: Bantam Books, 1968), p. 8.
11. K. H. Cooper, *The New Aerobics* (New York: Bantam Books, 1972), p. 38.
12. *Aerobics,* op. cit., p. 13.
13. P. O. Astrand, *Health and Fitness* (Ottawa: Information Canada, 1975), p. 25.